1-Day Diet
The Fastest Diet in the World

Jennifer Jolan
and
Rich Bryda

FACEBOOK

If you want to stay in touch and see what we're up to, join us here:
• www.facebook.com/10HourCoffeeDiet

Jennifer Jolan & Rich Bryda

COPYRIGHT AND TRADEMARK NOTICES

TABLE OF CONTENTS

Section 1: The 1-Day Diet, the Fastest "Diet" in the World   3

Bonus: 7 Special Weight Loss & Health "Helpers"   5

1   Introduction   15

2   Background Info about The 1-Day Diet Plan   21

3   Variations on a Theme – Choose the Best 1-Day Diet Plan for You   27

4   1-Day Diet Plan Costs   31

5   1-Day Diet Enhancer Tricks   35

6   Eating On Non-Diet Days With Some Gotchas   43

7   1-Day Diet Plan Q&A's   49

8   How Exercise Fits Into The 1-Day Diet Plan   53

9   Recap   55

Section 2: The 5:2 Diet Cheat Sheet: Breakthrough 2-Days-a-Week Dieting   57

10   Introducing the 5:2 Diet Cheat Sheet   59

11   Making the 5:2 Diet's "2" Much Better   63

12   The Science Behind I.F.   73

13   5:2 Fat-Burning - Inexpensive and Customizable   81

14   Making the 5:2 Diet Even Easier!   85

Section 3: STUPID Hormones! The Hormone Weight Loss Solution - Fix Your CRAZY Hormones and Finally Lose Weight for Good!   91

15   Introduction to Hormones and Health   93

16   Health is the Key, Not Weight   95

17   What Exactly is a Hormone?   99

18   Food and Hormones   103

19   A Healthy Hormone Diet   109

20   The Master Control Hormone   119

21   The Fat-Storing Hormone   123

22   The Fat-Removing and the "I Feel Full" Hormones   127

23   The Growing Up Healthy Hormone   131

24 Up and Downs: The Sleep and Stress Hormones   135
25 The Hunger-Stimulating and Rebuilding Hormones   139
26 The Sex-Related Hormones   145
27 The Adrenaline and the Fight or Flight Hormones   157
28 Hormone Summary   161
29 1-Day Diet Conclusion   163
    Bonus Gifts!   165
    References   167

Section 1:

The 1-Day Diet
The Fastest "Diet"
in the World!

1
7 SPECIAL WEIGHT LOSS & HEALTH "HELPERS"

Before getting to the 1-Day Diet we wanted to share some bonus tips that don't quite fit anywhere else in the book. These tips have to do with exercise and detoxing. Our *Running Sucks* book is where we go in depth and give you a complete program in regards to exercise and other non-diet related ways to lose weight and burn calories.

You can do most of those exercises in your home and finish them in five minutes or less. There's no point wasting hours of your time each week for minimal results when you can get better results in five minutes *at home*.

With the 1-Day Diet, you don't "need" to exercise more or even exercise at all to lose weight. But of course, exercise certainly would help with weight loss. So with all that said, we'll get to the tips.

I have a quick question I want you to answer.

Which of the following would you least want to lose?

    A. Your cell phone

    B. Your car

    C. Your house

    D. Your job

    E. Your TV

F. Your computer

G. Your body

If you answered G, Your Body – which you should have answered, then why do you treat your car, house, TV, computer, cell phone, and just about everything else better than you treat your own body?!

Starting right now, take responsibility for how you look and how you feel. Deliberately make choices that don't *contribute* to destroying your body.

Here are the 7 special weight loss and health "helpers":

The *Proper* Way to Breathe

Most people don't realize that their shallow breathing contributes to poor health through stagnant blood and lymphatic flow. Deep breathing oxygenates the blood and accelerates movement of your lymphatic fluids. By oxygenating your blood through deep breathing, you are actually creating energy for yourself. By breaking up stagnant blood flow, your blood will efficiently bring energy, essential nutrients, and hormones to every area of your body.

Just five to ten minutes a day of deep breathing will effectively prevent most sicknesses.

Deep breathing also helps your blood carry off toxins and excess fats floating in your bloodstream. It does this *while* speeding up your metabolism. Deep breathing isn't a "pure" weight loss technique, but it does contribute to weight loss. It also aids your body in getting rid of fat more efficiently. Deep breathing is one of the quickest ways to increase your energy levels and hardly anybody complains of having too much energy.

Here's how you best accomplish deep breathing:

Take a deep breath. Inhale strongly from your belly, not your chest. Inhale for five seconds. Hold it for five seconds. (Inhale from your nose and hold in your mouth.) Then after that, exhale for five seconds. Exhale from your mouth by slightly opening up your mouth. Don't cheat the time because you are only cheating yourself if you do. If you're going to cheat and not do it as outlined, don't even bother doing deep breathing.

Within a few days, your head and body will feel lighter, clearer, and more energetic. This is because you're getting more oxygen in your blood thanks to deep breathing.

Here's an easy way to remember it... 5-5-5-5.

Inhale for 5 seconds.

Hold in your mouth for 5 seconds.

Exhale for 5 seconds.

Do this deep breathing for 5 minutes a day.

Cold Water Treading – At Home!

Cold water, hot water, steam, and ice all produce different reactions from your body and your internal organs. For our purposes, we'll concentrate on cold water because it's considered "alive" as opposed to hot water, which is considered "dead."

Cold water energizes, invigorates, and fortifies the body. Cold water creates circulation and overcomes sluggishness while unblocking any energy barriers within your body. One of the reasons cold water works so great is because it stimulates the body into a reaction. I'll explain this further shortly when we talk about the details of cold water treading.

Cold water treading literally turns your body into a fat burning machine. The reason is simple. The cold water stimulates your body to heat up. Your body raises its core temperature as a reaction to the cold water, which is in effect forcing your body to a lower core temperature.

Think of your natural reaction when you're cold. You shiver. That's your body's way of creating heat to warm you up. This is very similar in nature. It's basically a fight between cold water and your body. Your body is saying "Uh, *nooooooo*, I'm going to internally heat up to fight you. I won't allow you to change the core temperature."

You can take advantage of this bodily reaction to cold water. Here is how you do cold water treading to force your body into a higher internal temperature that helps burn fat better.

Note: This is possible only if you have a tub/shower combo.

Simply take your normal shower. Once you finish, plug the bathtub up while turning the water to as cold as possible. Once you get about 3 inches of really cold water, stop the water and start walking in place in your cold water.

This is cold water treading. Do this for three minutes after your shower.

Now, I'm going to tell you something that is even better for fat loss and general health. Mentally, it's harder, but the results are even better: Take a cold shower… *I mean a real cold shower.* The shower should be so cold that you have a hard time breathing. Every second feels like a minute.

Cold showers are better than cold water treading for general health and weight loss since the cold water covers your whole body and not just your feet and lower legs. However, most people won't do them. Personally, I *don't* do cold water treading simply because cold showers are better and easier to do. But I'm realistic and know most people won't do cold showers, so I have a compromise that works great.

This is exactly what I do. I take my normal shower with the water slightly colder than I prefer. After I'm done with that, I turn the water to as cold as possible and let it spray all over my body for 20 seconds. That's it. Just 20 seconds.

After that, I turn the water off and get a towel to dry off as quickly as possible!

Some days I just can't bring myself to do this. You know what I mean right? But I can consistently do this about four days a week, especially when it's not winter.

One thing to keep in mind is that once you do the cold shower (or cold water treading), do *not* use hot or warm water on your body for the next 20 minutes. You will be tempted!

But doing so just ruins everything. Give your body a chance to react to the cold. It is that reaction you need for a metabolism boost.

You're going to first yell and curse my name when you try the cold showers, but you will soon think I'm a genius once you see the results. Try them. See for yourself. It's 20 seconds of torture, but it's worth it.

Jumping A Special Way

Jumping on a mini-trampoline is not only a great exercise, but it's good for your cells. You can get a mini-trampoline (called a *rebounder*) at Walmart for under $50 (if you're not in North America, do a search on the internet of where you can get it).

The rebounder is great to jump on for two minutes here and there. Those two minutes of jumping add up. A great time to use this is during commercials while you're watching TV. I give you permission to watch TV for an hour; however, with your mini-trampoline in front of you!

During each commercial, I want you to jump on the mini-trampoline. At the end of an hour, you would have jumped on the trampoline for 15 to 20 minutes. Don't use the excuse that you don't have time to do this. And if you don't watch TV, I'm sure you can still find a couple of minutes here and there throughout the day to jump on the mini-trampoline at home.

Besides during commercials, I also jump on the mini-trampoline before and after going to the bathroom, while I'm cooking, and after I put laundry in the washing machine. That's just my routine. If you're watching your kids, you can do it with them. Take turns. They love it!

Come on… don't think of lame excuses on why you can't do this. It's simple and can be done in your home anytime you feel like it. Plus the rebounder is small and you can leave it in your living room.

Doing this helps maintain a "youthfulness" to your cells due to its effects on improving the lymphatic system and its circulation throughout your body.

Lowering Your Set Point – The Simple Way

You have a weight that your body is comfortable at. This is your body's "set point."

If you start to lose weight, your body tries to get you back up to the set point. What your body's set point is determines what your weight is. This is why people who lose weight almost always gain the weight back.

Fortunately, you can change your set point. In fact, your body is always adjusting its set point. Your body determines its set point by the foods you've eaten recently (the past few weeks) and how much physical activity you've had recently.

The best exercise to lower your body's set point is walking. If you walk 30 minutes a day for five days a week, your body will lower its set point. When it does that, it basically helps unlock the switch for you to lose weight.

When your weight is way above your set point, get walking. I know this is not a revolutionary tip, but it is something basic to consider. Not every tip has to be flashy and new to effectively work in improving your health and helping you to lose weight.

How You Can Burn 18% More Calories While Walking

This is simple and it combines two previous tips. Do deep breathing while you walk.

Here's how... while you walk, inhale for five seconds through your nose, hold it in for five seconds, and exhale through your mouth for five seconds. Do that about once for every minute you walk. That means for a 30-minute walk, you do your 5-5-5 deep breathing routine 30 times.

The combined deep breathing and walking will help you burn off 18% more calories than just the walk itself due to the increased oxygenation of your blood from the deep breathing.

Brushing More than Your Hair

Your skin is the largest organ you have. Something you probably didn't know is it releases about a pound of toxins *each day* from your body!

The problem is, sometimes your skin can't excrete these toxins efficiently due to clogged pores. Your pores can get clogged by makeup, dirt, pollution, dead skin cells, and excreted wastes. With clogged pores, your skin traps toxins inside your body.

A lot of times, this results in cellulite. Yes. The. Dreaded. Cellulite.

Obviously, we don't want that. One way to help eliminate the problem is through dry skin brushing.

Some of the many weight loss and body enhancement benefits of dry skin brushing include:

- Helping you get rid of 1 pound of toxins from your body each day (there's always a give and take with toxins coming in and going out no matter what you do)

- Reducing cellulite

- Stimulating blood and lymph flow

- Stimulating your nervous system and hormones

You'll want to pick a brush has natural fiber bristles and a long handle so you can reach all of your back.

The best time to do dry brushing is right before you take a shower. Start by brushing your feet and make sure to brush towards your heart. Then brush up your legs, over your stomach and then brush your back and butt. If you have cellulite on your butt, hips, and or thighs, then do the brushing a little longer on those areas.

Note: If you have a lot of cellulite and a lot of discipline, you can literally dissolve a lot of your cellulite by doing this dry brushing on your cellulite areas for 10 minutes a day for about two months.

Yeah, it'll take a while. But it's worth it!

After your butt and back, finish up by dry brushing your arms, shoulders, and breasts. Obviously you'll want to brush lightly on your breasts.

Total time: A minute or two. (You can also dry brush a minute here and there whenever you get the chance; like when watching TV... even if it's only your arms that you dry brush.)

Then take a shower.

There are so many important benefits to dry brushing that I hope you seriously do it every day. Who doesn't want to get rid of cellulite and toxins from their body!

Earthy and Good

Many detoxing methods and supplements remove specific toxins from specific areas of your body. This is fantastic because many toxins sink into your cells and need to be grabbed any means possible.

Still, for the most part, your body does a good job at detoxing itself. When you eliminate urine and waste, your body has placed toxins in that waste. This is a perfect avenue for toxin elimination.

When you breathe out, your mucous membranes secrete toxins that leave your body through your exhaled breath.

When you sweat, your sweat glands are secreting waste out from your skin's pores. Exercising will improve the flow of those toxins, both from your sweat glands and through your intensive breathing.

It turns out your skin is a major toxin remover. Not only do your sweat glands secrete toxins, but waste can leave any pore in your body. Cellular and other bodily waste is eliminated through your pores.

The Helpful Clay

As you can see, without doing anything you are a detoxing machine. The problem is that depending on your lifestyle and the food you eat, the toxins catch up to you. Even before the somewhat dangerous and low-nutrient modern-day food supplies, and before the industrial revolution added pollutants into the air, and before plastics, pesticides, and other containments entered our water supply, our bodies would still get sick every year or so to perform an extra-powerful detox.

But today's world we're getting bombarded with toxins to the point that bodies can't keep up with the routine removal of environmental toxins that enter our systems.

Some of the symptoms of routine toxicity are:

- Mental dullness

- Aching-stiff joints

- Gas and bloat

- High acidity

- Digestive problems with the stomach and colon

- Acid reflux

- Fatigue

Let's get back to our skin. You might already know that your skin is the largest organ. The reason it's large is not due to its thickness but to its surface area. Throughout our skin on every part of our bodies are pores that help keep us as clean as they can. And we can tap into those pores to enable even more toxins to leave through our pores through the use of clay, *bentonite clay* to be specific.

More specifically known as *Calcium Bentonite Clay* therapy, the application of bentonite clay is one of the least invasive and safest means to detox that has been found. Plus, bentonite clay has a high negative ionic charge and is highly effective in pulling the toxins out from your skin like a magnet pulls metal filings.

Clay is alkaline-based, whereas we typically consume far too many acidic substances in our diets and on our skin. So after bentonite clay therapy, our skin not only has released extra toxins over the amount it released by itself, but our skin feels nice and clean afterwards and leaves us often feeling refreshed. The clay's alkaline property works to balance our skin.

Note: Clay is often used for acne treatment and radiation exposure.

Detoxing through the use of clay is nothing new. As a matter of fact, it may be one of the oldest detoxing methods known to man. Indigenous tribes have been using clay for skin therapy for thousands of years.

Clay as a Catalyst

As well as clay works on our skin, bentonite clay is also taken internally.

Both on our skin and when we consume it internally, clay is a catalyst. By that I mean it becomes active in the removal process of toxins from our bodies. Technically, a catalyst boosts chemical reactions and does so efficiently. Clay's catalyst action is so efficient it can remove toxins from our lower colons before they enter our bloodstream. This frees up nutrients to repair and revitalize our bodies.

In addition to its detoxing benefits, is clay actually the foundation of eternal youth too? Dr. Alexis Carrel of the Rockefeller Institute for Medical Research seems to think so based on his experiments from way back to the 1900's. *Years to Your Health* explained Dr. Carrel's study this way:

"He managed to sustain the life of cells from a chicken embryo by immersing the cells in a solution

containing all the nutrients necessary for life and changing the solution daily. The cells took up nutrients from the nutrient-rich broth and excreted their wastes into the same solution. The only thing Dr. Carrel did each day was discard the old solution and replace it with fresh nutrient solution. The chicken cells lived for 29 years until one night Dr. Carrel's assistant forgot to change the polluted solution! We do not know how much longer the cell's life could have been maintained. Dr. Carrel concluded at the end of his experiment that the cell is actually immortal. It is merely the fluid in which it floats which degenerates. He is quoted saying 'The cell is immortal. Renew this fluid at intervals, give the cell something on which to feed and, so far as we know, the pulsation of life may go on forever.' The average chicken lives about 7 years. His detoxified, properly nourished chicken cell lived for 29 years."

The upshot was that Dr. Carrel believed we don't get old because of time. Instead, we get old due to toxin build-up at the cell level. As it builds and our bodies cannot keep up, cell breakdowns begin to occur that overall we see as the effects of aging.

The Clay Therapy

Ran Knishinsky, author of The Clay Cure, is an advocate of eating or drinking clay daily. He states some of the benefits reported by people using liquid clay for a period of two to four weeks include:

- Improved intestinal regularity

- Relief from chronic constipation

- Diarrhea, indigestion

- Ulcers

- A surge in physical energy

- Clearer complexion

- Brighter, whiter eyes

- Enhanced alertness

- Emotional uplift

- Improved tissue and gum repair

- and increased resistance to infections.

Clay works on the entire organism. No part of the body is left untouched by its healing energies.

AboutClay.com suggests taking clay daily to maintain a good, clean digestive system. For adults, a normal dosage would be to take one to two ounces daily. When taking clay internally, keep your body hydrated by drinking eight to ten glasses of filtered, non-chlorinated, non-fluoridated water daily. The water helps to soften and loosen impacted fecal material lining the walls of your small intestine and colon. This material is then absorbed by the clay and removed from the body through normal elimination.

> Note: For an initial detox, take a higher dosage as follows: three ounces three times a day for four to six weeks and then gradually reduce to one to two ounces daily for maintenance.

One of the best clays available is Great Plains Bentonite Clay. You can find it on Amazon here:

http://www.amazon.com/Yerba-Prima-Bentonite-Detox-Ounce/dp/B00016XI7A

For using clay on your skin, you should look into clay baths. These are highly beneficial for detoxification, especially for cases of heavy metal poisoning. A typical clay bath would involve using a couple of cups of powdered clay in a bathtub and then run *very hot water* over the clay, as hot as it gets. Use a whisk to stir the clay around and to help it dissolve. When you've got about 3 inches of water in the tub and the clay is dissolved, start adding cooler water until the water reaches the desired temperature.

The bath should neither be too hot nor too cool, just nice, warm, and comfortable. Bathing time depends upon your condition, but can be anywhere from 10 to 20 minutes at the most. If you stay in too long you may have what is known as a *cleansing reaction* and can experience fatigue, headaches, muscle soreness, and so on. If this happens to you, note how long you were in the bath and spend half that time the next session.

Here's a good bentonite clay that you can purchase in bulk on Amazon here:

http://www.amazon.com/Frontier-Bulk-Bentonite-Powder-package/dp/B000UY8738

While doing the 1-Day Diet, consider using as many of the preceding 7 special weight loss and health "helpers" as possible.

OK. Now, what you've been waiting for... the 1-Day Diet.

1
INTRODUCTION

Welcome to the 1-Day Diet Plan. This may be one of those rare life-changing moments in your life. One that turns the tide on weight problems you may have had for a long time. This may be the turning point that turns your thighs and hips into lean, mean, sexy machines!

I believe when you finish the 1-Day Diet Plan, you will agree you've made a smart buying decision.

Why This Book Exists

I developed this book because so many diets out there don't work or simply aren't practical to do. The fact is most people won't stay on a diet very long when they feel deprived, like they're suffering, and or if they don't see fast results. Calorie-reduced diets eventually seem to create an insatiable feeding frenzy in most of us because we are not made to live for long with severe calorie restriction. Our body's defense mechanisms step in and take over.

Other diet plans are considered by a fair number of people to be unhealthy, such as the Pritikin diet that is said to raise our blood sugar to high levels at almost every meal and sacrifices healthy bones and muscles along the way.

Plus, let's face it. A diet is one of the hardest things we ever try to do. It isn't easy. We hear the following: "Your daily eating should be healthy; one that is more of a lifestyle than a diet. A lifestyle you can stick with forever." Yes, we hear those words, but they rarely sink in. So, it's on-again, off-again, and the pounds yo-yo, but always seem to yo-yo on the upside eventually.

The 1-Day Diet Plan solves all of that for you.

The 1-Day Diet Plan is a plan you *can* stick with and incorporate into the rest of your life... on and off at your convenience.

The Difficulty Factor

I want to assure you that you not only will lose a lot of weight fast (and *safely*) with this program, but you will also see a dramatic improvement in your health at the same time. The biggest bonus: the 1-Day Diet Plan is not difficult at all.

One of the primary reasons the 1-Day Diet Plan is so successful is that you get to continue eating your favorite foods, if you want. You should never feel deprived. Never will you feel as though you're suffering. Yes, it sounds great doesn't it? When you see how the 1-Day Diet Plan operates, you'll understand how I can make these bold claims. And you'll also realize it has the complete ring of truth because it is true.

With the information in this book, you will never need to buy another diet program or hyped-up, expensive weight loss pill again if you don't want to. If you find yourself on the scales upswing, you can hop right back on the 1-Day Diet whenever you feel like it… at your convenience… and for the rest of your life. This is why it's both a lifestyle *and* a temporary diet – the best of both worlds!

Other Plans

Feel free to learn other things about weight loss and dieting if you want. However, other information would be considered a "side dish" as compared to the 1-Day Diet Plan being your "main course." Side dishes are nice, but they're not necessary.

They're complimentary.

Over the course of this book, I am going to reveal to you a very powerful and proven system… yet it's very easy and practical. We designed the 1-Day Diet plan to include great flexibility as to how you implement it.

For an initial period, however, I urge you to strictly follow what I say to do. Do exactly as I say for the first 4 weeks. The good thing about this requirement is, as I said before, the 1-Day Diet Plan is simple to follow.

Why Four Weeks?

Many diets have an initial requirement period. For example, the Atkins Diet requires that you stick to proteins and virtually no carbohydrates for the first several days. Others require this also.

But my reason for requiring that you follow the 1-Day Diet Plan for four weeks is different from the rest. Why? I want you to follow what I say because I want you to prove to yourself, without a doubt, that the 1-Day Diet Plan works before allowing yourself to give yourself more freedom and flexibility to make "little" changes to it.

Note: Keep this in mind. Four weeks isn't long at all. In four weeks from today, guess what? You will either be four weeks older *and* will be astounded at the results you see from the ultra-simple 1-Day Diet Plan *or* you will be four weeks older and still looking the same and weighing the same... or more... if you choose not to follow the 1-Day Diet Plan as it is outlined for you to be successful. The four weeks are going to pass anyway. Why not make the most of them?

Once you gain incredible confidence in knowing the 1-Day Diet Plan works, you can then make reasonable changes based on your experience with doing it. You *can* customize the 1-Day Diet Plan the way you want to do it.

By doing it the way I ask, four weeks, and then you follow it the way *you want,* you'll see that the 1-Day Diet Plan becomes a diet you can rely on for the rest of your life.

You can keep going back to it again and again whenever you gain a few pounds and want to lose them quickly.

How Much Weight Can You Lose?

This is the good part!

You are probably interested in how much weight you'll lose and how quickly those fat pounds will disappear.

Here's a simple rule of thumb:

The average person who is 30 or more pounds overweight, who follows the 1-Day Diet Plan, can expect a two to five pound weight loss upon waking up the day after doing the diet *the first time*!

So, you will weigh yourself right before you go to bed *the night before or the morning* you start the 1-Day Diet Plan. You then will weigh yourself again *the morning after* the 1-Day Diet Plan... immediately after awakening, going to the bathroom, but before you drink anything or eat breakfast.

Now, I don't want you to use the first day's weight loss as a basis on the success and effectiveness of the system. *Don't get hung up on that initial weight loss.*

Note: You should not monitor your weight constantly for a variety of reasons we'll talk about throughout this book. Psychologically weighing yourself every day or two can be discouraging since weight loss doesn't happen in a fixed amount each day. More important, your *fat* is what you want to lose, not muscle mass. You will see more below that the 1-Day Diet Plan is great for keeping your lean muscle mass and dropping the fat. It may even increase your lean muscle mass, thus increasing your weight. Lost pounds are not important... lost *fat* is important![1]

About that daily weight loss: weight loss is not linear, meaning it's not straight down.

There are natural ups and downs based on a lot of factors. People are surprised on any weight management plan to find that some weeks nothing goes away and others a significant number of pounds just disappear in a 24-hour period. Our bodies regulate our weight and fat loss more than we give them credit for. Hormones often determine when fat increases or decreases.

Also, some of your weight that you lose will be "water weight" and you will in fact gain some of it back. This is normal and natural. *Don't worry* about that. Keep in mind that you'll be losing fat. Over time you'll also lose all your unnecessary water bloat too.

Note: Your body is made up of over 70% water. This is why you'll always have water weight fluctuations depending on the food you eat from one day to the next, the number and type of liquids you consume, the amount of exercise or physical work you do, and your hormones.

But to give you an even better idea of what to expect, over the first month of doing the 1-Day Diet Plan as I outline the plan, the average overweight person can lose up to 20 to 35 pounds doing the first version of this plan. The best part is this: the more overweight you are, the more weight you can expect to lose.

If you have less fat and weight to lose, then obviously you'll lose less weight overall… but you'll still almost instantly begin to lose whatever fat you do have, and quickly.

Clothes Tell the Tale – So Does Your Belly

Along with watching your weight on the scale, do these three things the first four weeks:

1. Pay attention to how your clothes fit around your waist.
2. Check how you look in the mirror. (This is the best part!)
3. Take your measurements.

Those three simple things give a more accurate picture of fat loss than simply looking at the scale. Scales don't always give the full picture, but taking your measurements and seeing the fat loss in the mirror along with how your clothes fit do tell a more complete picture in regards to how successful your weight loss is.

The 1-Day Diet Plan is especially good at eliminating the horrid *belly fat*. You'll see this is true from measurements and from the way your clothing fits. Scales won't tell you necessarily how much belly fat you're losing, *especially* if you're exercising and building some lean muscle mass too. In fact, the morning after *each* time you do the 1-Day Diet, you will notice your belly is leaner and tighter upon waking up.

If you have a lot of belly fat, the reduction may not be as visibly noticeable to you, but you can be sure your belly fat is getting whittled down fast.

It's a System to be Followed in Sequence

Before we get to the good stuff, the first big idea I want to share with you is that this plan is not just a book… *it is a system.*

The sequence you follow the 1-Day Diet is a very, very big deal.

I am going to show you step by step exactly how to lose a lot of weight, get healthier, and keep the weight off for the rest of your life. This is completely possible *without* depriving yourself of your favorite foods. If you follow the steps I lay out in the system, you will get the same or very similar results as the many other people who have succeeded with the 1-Day Diet before you. This includes professional athletes who rely on their bodies to earn millions of dollars.

Let me try that another way. Millionaire athletes trust various versions of this diet because it works. If it didn't work, it could possibly cost them millions of dollars.

Let's face it. You paid good money for this 1-Day Diet Plan and right now I'm about to show you what an incredibly smart decision you made. You will reap the benefits of this investment for years and years. This means a skinnier, happier, healthier, improved version of *you*.

You got this book because you want to lose weight by using a practical diet that is easy to do without having to suffer like you do on most diets. Judge the value of this information on four things and only these four things:

1. How much weight you lose using it.
2. How fast you're able to lose that weight.
3. How easy it was for you to lose that weight.
4. The amount of money you end up saving because you're using the 1-Day Diet Plan (and don't forget the money savings due to improved health and a lifetime of lower health care costs.)

That's it.

If I could help you lose over 20 pounds and it only took one page to do, would that not be very valuable in spite of it just being a page? I'd say so.

Judge the 1-Day Diet Plan by what the information does for you and the results you get. You want to look better and be more energetic by losing a lot of weight. If you listen to me, it's going to happen. I *promise* you that if you put your faith in me, and this information, I'm going to over-deliver beyond your wildest expectations.

A month from now, you will look in the mirror and be amazed at your weight loss transformation. And it won't be that difficult to accomplish. It will actually *be simple*. The result is that you won't be able to stop smiling and feeling great about yourself. In addition, your friends, relatives, and co-workers will be asking you how the heck you lost so much weight, so fast.

Right now you may not believe me.

You probably have some vague hope that I can help you, but you're not 100% convinced. That's fine. I'm used to skepticism because there is so much hype and misinformation in the weight loss industry. It's completely understandable.

As you read through the next few pages, you'll start believing in me and in the possibility that this truly will work for you. But the true test comes when you try out the 1-Day Diet Plan. This is where you can prove me wrong and make a liar out of me.

However, that won't happen.

Instead, a month from now after you've given my system an honest try, what will usually happen is you'll either email me to thank me or leave a review on Amazon thanking me and saying how happy you are. So, four weeks from now, I hope you send me an email letting me know how much weight you've lost or leave a review on Amazon.com.

Okay. It's time to get started.

2
BACKGROUND INFO ABOUT THE 1-DAY DIET PLAN

The basis of the 1-Day Diet Plan revolves around *intermittent fasting* (*IF*). Wait, wait, wait! Before you get any ideas, no, you *won't* starve.

The standard way of starving yourself and not eating anything on a fast doesn't work for long term weight loss because you end up like a yo-yo and the lost weight goes back on your thighs and hips and belly due to losing muscle and water weight. This is most common for diets that attack pounds and not specifically fat.

The reason why people gain the weight they lost back is because your muscles are more metabolically active than your fat. In other words, a pound of muscle burns far more calories each day than a pound of fat. This has to do with your basal metabolic rate (*BMR*).[2]

Calories Just to Live

Most of the calories and fat you burn throughout a normal day don't come from exercise. You actually burn very few calories during exercise. Fat is burned off more through the food you eat – and don't eat – than exercise. For proof, look up how many calories you burn watching an hour of TV on the couch and calories burned walking on a treadmill for an hour. The difference might make you sell your treadmill!

Most calories burned off each day are burned off simply to give you and your body the necessary fuel to survive. Not to be active, but simply to survive.

But, because your muscles require more calories to survive, they burn off more calories. So the more muscle you have on your body, the easier it is for you to lose weight and keep it off. This is why men usually have an easier time losing weight than women.

And this is why a starvation diet or fast is *not* good for weight loss… or your health.

When you're starving, your body eats your muscles for energy. When you lose muscle, you lose a key part in a fast metabolism that helps you burn off more calories each day (while doing nothing… just surviving). This is exactly what happens when you fast.

So Why Are We Going to Eat Like This?

Having said that fasting is bad for true fat-based weight loss, you'll wonder why I am recommending a form of fasting. The answer is simple; just like the 1-Day Diet Plan is simple. There's a way to lose a lot of fat while fasting and at the same time *preserve your muscles*. And the best part is that this kind of fasting does not involve you starving or even being hungry.

By doing this type of fasting, you unlock the power of fasting for weight loss because you don't hurt your metabolism. In other words you don't lose any muscle weight during the process. All the weight you lose will be fat and excess water bloat.

So, how do you do this?

A Very Special Kind of Eating Routine

An extremely special fast exists called intermittent fasting (IF). With IF, you will use small frequent doses of protein to preserve your muscles. This causes your body not to worry that it's starving and you don't suffer from the effects of starving on a normal fast.

There is something interesting about fasting.

Fasting has been known to provide several health, mental, life-extension, and even spiritual benefits for thousands of years. You've heard of people fasting for a day or more, sometimes even for a week or more. Several different kinds of fasts are possible including a food fast where you just drink liquids such as fruit juice. (I never suggest you do this.) Some fasts require that you eat nothing for one day and then eat regularly the next. Lots of fast options exist.[3]

The amazing thing is that it doesn't seem to matter *which* fast you do. Your body still appears to gain the health benefits (not necessarily the long term weight loss benefits, however) of fasting whether you fast straight through or break it up or fast just on liquids for a while! In other words, if you fasted for a week without food and only water, or you fasted only on water every other day for two weeks (a form of intermittent fasting), the end result appears to be the same! Your body's reaction appears to gain the same health benefits.

Note: For those who fast for spiritual reasons, you may not see the same mental or spiritual benefits from fasting intermittently as you do from a multi-day fast.

So, for those wanting the physical benefits of fasting, you don't have to worry about starving several days. We saw earlier that doing this greatly deteriorates your muscles by robbing your body of them in an effort to survive. Fasting off and on gives you the same physical benefits without the agony of going without food for several days in a row.

Dr. Joseph Mercola describes the result of one study on IF. He tells how a 2007 American Journal of Clinical Nutrition study divided the study's participants into two groups. Each group had the same volume and number of calories. In other words, they had identical diets during the study. The calories were ample to maintain their weight.

The only difference between the two groups is this:

- The first group ate their prescribed food in a typical three-meals-daily plan.
- The second group only ate within an eight-hour time frame each day.[4]

Get it? They ate the same food, but the second set of participants ate only within an 8-hour period and fasted for 16 hours.

The results are astounding:

Note: Normally when people perform this kind of intermittent fast, they eat between 12 noon and 8 at night. This means they skip breakfast. If you've heard the adage that breakfast is "the most important meal of the day," you've probably been told wrongly. During the night your body detoxes while you sleep. In the morning the reason you don't normally awaken famished and starving is because your body *continues to detox* for a few hours after waking up. By eating a breakfast (by *breaking fast* in other words), you interrupt that important detox routine that your body wants to do. Your body then tries to play catch-up and finish its detox, but bodily resources must be sent to digest your new food. The detox is far less efficient and you throw off fewer toxins and gain weight more easily.

Dr. Mercola concludes by showing those who ate the same calories in an IF routine had a significant change in fat mass. And it's the *fat mass* we don't want.

He states that intermittent fasting is attributed to many benefits including:

- The hormones insulin and leptin[5] being normalized which helps guard you against diabetes, heart disease, and even cancer.
- Ghrelin levels are normalized. Ghrelin[6] is the hormone of "hunger." When on any diet plan, your chance of failure is increased directly by how much higher the levels of hunger you have.
- HGH – the Human Growth Hormone[7] – is normalized. The HGH is vital for health, fitness, and staying young.
- Triglyceride levels[8] are lowered.
- Free radical[9] and inflammation[10] are lessened allowing your body to heal more rapidly when damaged or after exercise.

But *if* is even better when you do it the 1-Day Diet Plan way!

Note: Fasting of any kind is dependent on your lifestyle and goals. If you are a hardcore athlete, fasting will affect your performance, sometimes for good and sometimes not (not the best idea to fast right before competition). For most people who are not elite athletes, IF is extremely beneficial (it's beneficial for athletes also, but they need to be careful with timing their IF).

IF – The 1-Day Diet Plan Way!

Before showing you intermittent fasting as you'll do it on the 1-Day Diet Plan, I'm going to discuss something called *protein waters*. Don't confuse protein water with protein shakes or those meal replacement shakes.

Protein waters are the secret key to your weight loss success. Protein waters are the biggest breakthrough in dieting in the last fifteen or more years.

Keep in mind that the 1-Day Diet Plan isn't necessarily a lifelong endeavor. It is one of the few weight loss regimens you *can* leave and return to easily, as needed to adjust your fat loss.

What you're going to do on the 1-Day Diet Plan is easy to remember. And simplicity is the key to success on anything like weight loss. Nothing can be simpler than this:

On the 1-Day Diet, you will not eat any food whatsoever for one day.

Wait, stay with me here. This doesn't violate anything I said earlier about calorie-restrictive diets being bad. Plus, going a full day without eating anything is not nearly as bad as it sounds when you do it this way.

You won't feel as though you're suffering. I promise. Just follow the instructions I'm about to give to you and it'll be really easy. And the weight loss results will blow your mind.

Remember: I'm talking about possibly losing an easy 20+ pounds in the first month alone. Not only that, you can *still eat all your favorite foods. But...* you must eat them on the days between your protein water days.

The protein water days are the key and each of those days comprises what is known as the 1-Day Diet Plan.

The Plan

What you're going to do is drink seven to nine protein waters each day you do the 1-Day Diet Plan. Drink one about every 1.5 to 2.5 hours. Don't deviate from this plan the entire day.

These are *not* intended to be meal replacement protein shakes. They are nothing like that. These are not meant to fill you up completely.

What they are meant to do is key: preserve your muscle mass while making it so you don't feel like you're starving and suffering. It's actually quite pleasant. You'll find that out once you start doing the plan.

The Ingredients

The protein water is simply this:

1. Put 9 to 14 ounces of water in a cup, glass, water bottle, or jar.
2. Add 10 to 15 grams of protein.
3. Shake it or stir it.
4. Drink it all within five minutes.

Note: If each scoop of your protein powder has 24 grams of protein in it (this is common), you would use about a half scoop (or a little more) for each protein water you drink during the day.

And yes, that is it. That *is* the key to losing fat and preserving muscle mass (and your metabolism) without even the hunger pangs of a typical diet or fast.

Set a timer. Drink your protein water mixed as described above. Do so once every 1.5 to 2.5 hours. Fortunately, your cell phone will have a timer or alarm which makes it really simple to be reminded of when it's time for your next protein water.

I personally use canning jars made of glass. I also recommend you use small, plastic shaker bottles that you can find at any health food store. Be sure to get only BPA-free plastic shaker bottles. I like to make a few protein waters at one time (either the night before the 1 Day Diet or the morning of the diet) so I don't have to bother getting out the protein and making a new protein water every 1.5 to 2.5 hours. It's ok to pre-make them and leave in the fridge over night or during the day.

Do whatever works best for you.

I usually make the first four protein waters the night before I begin the 1-Day Diet Plan routine. I simply add about 10 ounces of filtered water to the canning jar and then add 10 to 15 grams of protein powder to it. Again, this is about a half scoop for the protein powder (I'll suggest the brand to get in a few moments... although pretty much all brands work fine as long as they fit in the nutritional guidelines).

I shake each of them up and put in the fridge and leave overnight.

When I wake up, I give it a quick shake and have my first protein water.

Then after that, I set the alarm on my cell phone to ring in 105 minutes. This is an hour and 45 minutes. When the alarm goes off, I have my next protein water. I keep doing that until all nine of my protein waters are finished for the day. You can also change up the amount of time between each protein water based on if you're a little bit hungry or whether you're not so hungry. Just fit each protein water into the 1.5 to 2.5-hour timeline.

Helpful Details

What we've found through trial and error and based off a lot of feedback is that seven to nine total protein waters during the day is ideal. Nine protein waters a day seems to get the best weight loss results (surprising to most people), but seven protein waters work fine and get great results too.

Just remember that you must time these so you have a protein water every 1.5 to 2.5 hours. Never drink one outside that time range! This timing has been tested and perfected to maintain muscle mass (and maintain your metabolism), to maximize fat loss, and to keep you from feeling hungry. You may feel some hunger the *first* day you start the 1-Day Diet Plan. That's fine. It's your body's way of adjusting. After that you should feel "empty" but not hungry on each protein water day you decide to do.

The next day after doing the 1-Day Diet, you should wake up and be a few pounds lighter.

Sequencing your 1-Day Diet every other day, or *at least* twice a week for a month, will lead to incredible weight loss for you. I strongly urge you to choose the every other day option.

For variety, I next want to provide some outlines for different options using the 1-Day Diet Plan.

3
VARIATIONS ON A THEME –
CHOOSE THE BEST 1-DAY DIET PLAN FOR YOU

I'm going to give you a few options. You can choose a 1-Day Diet plan that works best for you given your personal preferences and tastes. I suggest that you try following the first plan I offer as it provides the maximum benefit. But if you want to modify the details, the follow-up variations may be better for you.

1-Day Diet Plan #1: Lose Up to 20+ Pounds in the First Month

This plan revolves around using the 1-Day Diet Plan protein waters every other day for a month. So, you'll follow the plan about 15 total days in the month.

If you want to lose a lot of weight *fast*, this is the plan to start with. The average range of weight loss is between 20 to 35 pounds for overweight people who have done this.

Now to be clear, yes the people who lose around 35 pounds on this are the ones who are 100+ pounds overweight and are dedicated. The more obese you are, the more weight you will lose.

But if that doesn't apply to you, it doesn't matter. If you are not that obese, losing 35 pounds in a month would be too quick of a weight loss anyway and could be unhealthy. Your body will know how to react properly to the 1-Day Diet Plan. Let your body do its thing. Fortunately, your body does want to drop fat on the plan. Let your body do what it wants to do. So if you have 10 pounds to lose, you won't lose 35 pounds. You simply don't have 35 pounds of excess weight to lose.

But you should lose all 10 of those pounds. And the best news is that it probably won't take you the full month to lose them. This every-other-day plan is the one I want you to start on regardless of how much weight you want to lose and how fast you want to lose it. I need you to learn and see firsthand the power of this dieting protocol. I need you to develop a confidence and faith that this can and does work for you.

Once you develop this confidence in the diet, you can always come back to the 1-Day Diet Plan months or years from now and do it again if you ever regain some fat weight. I never expect you to do these protein waters every other day for the rest of your life. Not even twice a week for the rest of your life.

My Personal Regimen Should Be Good for You

In spite of me being at my ideal weight, I follow the 1-Day Diet Plan protein waters once a week, every week for the health and cleansing benefits. Given what I said earlier about IF, you know that fasting one day a week for several weeks can offer virtually the same benefits as fasting several days in a row. Only it's much easier to follow the plan one day a week and the protein waters help ensure fat loss while telling your body it's safe to keep the muscle mass (so your metabolism doesn't down-regulate and slow down).

The once a week 1-Day Diet Plan protein waters also help me to maintain my ideal weight while allowing me to eat like a normal person the six other days each week. Actually, I should modify that statement. Even though I can, and do, eat "like a normal person" those 6 other days, I'm usually following my 10-Hour Coffee Diet those days.

I will talk about the once a week 1-Day Diet Plan shortly.

First, I want to say one more thing about your weight loss. I only give you the range of weight loss for the first month because after that it's hard to quantify the weight loss and make it relevant to each person individually.

In essence, the amount of weight loss is most correlated to the amount of weight you need to lose. The more overweight you are; the more weight you will lose. I have to harp on that point just to be clear.

After that first month of losing a lot of weight, it's nearly impossible to even guess or estimate how much weight you will lose moving forward. Your body will wax and wane and drop unexpectedly on some weeks and stay the same others.

It's all over the place for people. But our bodies know what to do as long as we fuel them properly.

I will state clearly that the 1-Day Diet Plan will work for as long as you need to lose weight.

1-Day Diet Plan #2: Lose Up to 15 Pounds in the First Month

If you're not able to do the 1-Day Diet Plan every other day, you can do it twice a week and still lose a lot of weight.

If you start on this program, the first month you should lose around 15 pounds (if you have a lot of weight to lose).

I suggest that you drink the protein waters on Mondays and Thursdays if you choose this version. But that's not set in stone. Do whatever works best for *you*. The main thing is to put two to three days between each 1-Day Diet Plan protein water day if you don't follow the every-other day routine the first month.

> **Note:** If you're really busy at work and it's kind of inconvenient to do the protein waters there, make it so one of the 1-Day Diet Plan protein water days is on a day off.

These weight loss results are also incredible. Just follow the 1-Day Diet Plan for one day and see how it goes. After that, decide between doing it every other day and twice a week (you could also do it three times a week as a middle-ground).

1-Day Diet Plan #3: Never Get Fat Again

This plan is for when you pretty much lost all the weight you need to lose. Think about your past with diets. If you are like most people, it wasn't the diet that was the problem as much as the weight gained following the diet. This is the common problem. Literally, if you don't consider any eating plan a lifelong habit, you will always think in short run concepts and in the long run you will almost surely revert back to the weight gain.

It's not you; it's *all of us* who do not follow a life-long eating regimen.

But even following a life-long regimen isn't enough because we age, our bodies change, our metabolisms change as we age, our hormones naturally change, and the battle of the bulge does get more difficult as the years pass.

Wouldn't it be wonderful if the invariable fat gain never occurs? You now have the tool to make sure!

Once you achieve your optimal weight, you can switch to following the 1-Day Diet Plan's protein waters once a week. Or, you can do them whenever you've regained a few pounds that you want to lose quickly.

This plan is more for your lifelong weight maintenance. Still, it's quite possible to consistently lose weight on this version of the 1-Day Diet as well. You'll usually end up losing two to five pounds each time you follow this plan.

If You Don't Do This Weekly, There's *Still* An Answer!

But, if you don't do the 1-Day Diet Plan at least once a week, there's a good chance you'll fall back to unhealthy eating habits and regain weight.

That's fine. For maybe the first time in your life, regaining some fat is not the problem it once was.

You *don't* need to do the 1-Day Diet every week. I'm just saying that if you don't do this once a week, there's a chance you'll regain weight. And if and when that happens, you can quickly lose that weight by doing the 1-Day Diet Plan once or twice again.

Then you can go back to not doing it for however long.

Basically, with this plan you can eat like a normal person until eating like a normal person (eating bad foods) gets you to the point that you gained some weight and you need to do something about it.

So, that's when you do something about it.

You do the 1-Day Diet Plan to lose the weight. That's what makes the 1-Day Diet Plan so great. You don't always have to do it. You just do it when you have to do it… when you need to lose some weight. You can fall back to it. It is old reliable. It is always there for you.

In spite of being able to return to the plan anytime you want or need to, I do encourage you to follow the 1-Day Diet Plan at least once a week just to make it easy to stay at your ideal weight and because of the powerful health benefits of the 1-Day Diet Plan. When you don't eat food for the day and you're only drinking protein waters, your body naturally begins a process of detoxing and cleansing during the break you're giving to your digestive system. You're also training your body to be more insulin sensitive,[11] which helps you to ward off type 2 diabetes.[12]

But, if you want to stop doing the 1-Day Diet Plan for a few months or you simply forget to do it for a few months... that is fine too.

Just know that you can always fall back to the 1-Day Diet Plan as a guaranteed way to lose any extra weight that you have.

4
1-DAY DIET PLAN COSTS

If you're unfamiliar with protein powders and their costs, here's the cost breakdown for following the 1-Day Diet Plan on the protein waters days only.

I'm not counting your normal food days because I don't know what you normally eat.

If you want to figure out your cost savings for each day you're on the 1-Day Diet Plan, then just figure out how much your normal food and drink costs are on the days you eat and drink like normal. Then subtract the costs of the 1-Day Diet Plan from that. Those are your savings for each day.

Figuring the Costs

For the every other day 1-Day Diet Plan you will do a total of 15 days of protein waters in a month.

I can only use the cost of the protein powder that I use as an example. What you use may be more expensive. I've used a bunch of different protein powders to test out their effectiveness and I've had a lot of feedback from others who have tested out various protein powders.

The key about buying a protein powder for this is to buy a whey protein powder that has 20+ grams of protein and fewer than five grams of fat and carbohydrates in each serving.

The brand of protein powder that I use is called Optimum Nutrition 100% Whey Gold

Standard. It's 5 pounds and costs about $53 (as of the time I write this) on Amazon at this link:

http://www.amazon.com/Optimum-Nutrition-Standard-Double-Chocolate/dp/B000QSNYGI

I personally like the chocolate mint, banana cream, and the delicious strawberry flavors. Choose whichever flavor you think you'll like the most. If you're a big coffee drinker, you may want the mocha cappuccino flavor (especially since you can't drink coffee on the protein water days). You should take a look at my book, *The 10-Hour Coffee Diet*,[13] if you're big into coffee.

The flavors vary a little on their servings, but as I write this now you will get around 77 serving with 24 grams of protein per serving. That's a total of 1,848 grams of protein per five-pound jug.

If you take 10 grams of protein for each protein water (a little less than a half scoop for this particular protein powder), a single container should last you 184 total protein waters. This means that if you have 9 protein waters a day (you may have as few as 7 protein waters a day… figure out what works best for you), this will last you about 20 days' worth of protein waters on the 1-Day Diet Plan (184 divided by 9).

Since you're doing these protein waters every other day (hopefully), a jug that costs $53 will last you 40 days… or almost 6 weeks. But we'll calculate costs based on the actual days you used the protein powder.

$53 divided by 20 days = $2.65 a day for each day you're on the 1-Day Diet Plan.

If you were to use 7 protein waters a day (10 grams each protein water, or 70 grams of protein per day), the total amount of days on the 1-Day Diet Plan for this jug of protein powder that I use would be almost 26 days (184 divided by 7).

The total daily cost of each day on the 1-Day Diet Plan (not counting your normal food eating days) is about $2 a day ($53 divided by 26 days).

So, since you're doing the 1-Day Diet Plan protein waters every other day, the *Optimum Nutrition* protein powder that costs $53 at Amazon would last you 52 days (almost 8 weeks) until you needed to buy another one.

Since most people will lose so much weight in the first month of doing the diet every other day (15 times in 1 month), you'll probably be able to cut back from the every other day pace.

Instead of doing it every other day, with all the weight you will have lost after the first month, you may only need to do it once or twice a week during the second month. So in fact, this one jug of protein powder would actually last even longer than 52 days for you.

The cost savings are obviously *substantial*. You'll save a lot of money!

For people not in the USA, the brand of protein powder doesn't seem to be a big factor in the success of this plan as long as you use a quality brand and make sure it has the right ratio of protein to carbs and fat in it.

I've used GNC's *100% Whey Banana Cream* flavor and that worked great. I also used Walmart's cheap protein powder and that also worked fine.

About the Protein

The feedback I've gotten back from all the testers who used all different kinds of protein powder shows that the protein powder you use doesn't really matter as long as it is a decent quality protein (whey protein powders seem to work best, but you can also use hemp, pea, or egg protein powders as well and you'll be fine. But know they are much more expensive and usually don't have the correct ratio between protein and carbs/fat).

Note that I didn't include the costs of the diet enhancers (I'll talk about those shortly) into total cost. If you wanted to factor those in, the 1-Day Diet Plan would end up costing about $3 a day. Still, I think you see that you'll save a ton of money while losing weight and getting healthier at the same time.

If you can't find a protein powder that is as cheap as the one I buy, then your costs will be more per day, but still ridiculously cheap. Don't worry if you spend more than $53 for a protein powder. It lasts many days and you *will* save money doing this diet.

Whatever protein powder you buy, you can do the same calculations I just did above and you'll see that you'll still save a lot of money regardless of the protein powder chosen. Again, add up the costs of your food and drinks and compare it to the costs of these protein waters. Even with a more expensive protein powder, you still save a lot of money.

Note: If you go to Starbucks, a coffee alone costs more than $3!

So, one Starbucks coffee costs more than being on the 1-Day Diet Plan for an entire day.

With the economy and healthcare system the way it is these days (not good and getting worse), this diet offers a great combination of weight loss, saving money, and improving your overall health. The more often you do the 1-Day Diet Plan each month (up to 15 times a month maximum), the more money you save.

Keep these cost savings in mind because other diets will cost you extra money instead of saving you money. In addition, they those diets don't work as effectively and aren't as easy to stick to because you're required to do them daily.

With the 1-Day Diet, you get breaks. You take a break at least every other day, or more depending on which routine you follow. This makes adhering to the diet much easier over the long run.

That is a big key as to whether you're successful or not with a diet: The sticking-with-it factor.

One last thing... sometimes people hit a wall in the late afternoon or early evening and feel the need to eat. That happens sometimes. No problem. Don't make a habit of it, but you can break off the diet and eat dinner. If you get hungry after dinner, then just have another protein water.

If you do break off the diet for an evening meal, you can then do the 1-Day Diet the next day starting fresh. And don't be surprised if you wake up lighter the next day even after eating dinner!

5
1-DAY DIET ENHANCER TRICKS

I'm going to share with you some things you can use to enhance the 1-Day Diet Plan weight loss results and make it mentally easier to get through the day you're using just protein waters and not eating anything… and not drinking anything other than water between each protein water.

All of these bonus enhancers are cheap. And as I showed you in the previous section above, the 1-Day Diet Plan is already extremely cheap to do.

The Five Diet Enhancers

Below are five diet enhancers you can use and why you may want to use them.

Our First Diet Enhancer

L-Tyrosine[14] is a pre-cursor to the brain neurotransmitters dopamine and norepinephrine. L-Tyrosine helps to elevate your mood and make you feel good. It makes it mentally and emotionally easier to deal with not being able to eat any food on the 1-Day Diet Plan days.

Although you usually won't feel hungry while on the plan, there will be points during the day where you may want to eat food out of habit. L-Tyrosine will help blunt your mental and emotional need of food.

I suggest you take L-Tyrosine with either your first or second protein water of the day (between protein waters would be even better, if possible). Take three grams, which is six pills (pills are usually 500mg each).

If you're in the USA or Canada, you can buy L-Tyrosine at Amazon or at this link:

http://www.bodybuilding.com/store/now/lty.html

120 capsules cost under $8 (as I write this). So if you take 6 capsules a day, it will take 20 days to use up the bottle.

Note: If you're doing the 1-Day Diet Plan every other day and take the 6 capsules only on the 1-Day Diet Plan days and not on the food days, it will last 40 total days.

I recommend L-Tyrosine highly. It puts you in a good mood while on the protein water days because it naturally elevates a person's mood. It also helps to blunt possible headaches you may get the first one or two protein water days due to a lack of caffeine or sugar (caffeine or sugar withdrawal symptoms).

If you're not in the USA or Canada, check your local health food stores or search online for L-Tyrosine.

Green Tea

Green tea by itself is excellent for long-term health and weight loss. Green tea also helps to burn fat and increases your metabolism.

The polyphenols in green tea help activate the enzymes that are responsible for burning off fat by dissolving excess triglycerides. The *epigallocatechin gallate* (EGCG)[15] in green tea stimulates the metabolism and accelerates weight loss.

So, what you want to do is buy a box of green tea from your grocery store. I personally buy a box of 20 tea bags of Carrington Green Tea from Walmart for about $1 (as I write this... prices on everything seem to be increasing all the time lately).

To use them, I boil about 30 ounces of water. Once the water starts to boil, I take it off the stove and pour it into 3 canning jars that are made of glass. Each canning jar can hold about 30 ounces of liquid, but pour just 10 or so ounces into each.

Each canning jar already has 1 green tea bag in it.

I let the green tea steep in the hot water for about 10 minutes and then take out the tea bags. Then I put the 3 canning jars in the fridge to let them cool off overnight. I make this batch of tea the night before I plan to follow the 1-Day Diet Plan.

Then the next day with the green tea cold, those 3 green teas will comprise my first 3 protein waters. All I have to do is add 10-15 grams of protein to it, shake, and it's ready.

Essentially they are now *green tea protein waters.*

Note: You can't drink these "green tea protein waters" hot. They have to be cool or you'll slightly degrade the protein.

I do it the night before, but you can make the green tea whenever you like. Just make sure it's cold to drink. (If you want, you can drink green tea or any other type of tea (hot or cold) between protein waters. They won't interfere with your weight loss results.) I'm referring to tea that uses tea bags, not tea or green tea in a bottle at the store.

One thing I want to make clear. Please try to avoid putting hot water in any type of plastic container, including shaker bottles. The reason is because the hot water activates the Xenoestrogens[16] in the plastics and they will leech into the water. That's bad. Xenoestrogens will mess up your hormones.

So, when making the green tea, please use a glass container or containers to avoid Xenoestrogens. You can find BPA-free containers,[17] but glass is just simpler and ensures, hot or cold, you won't be getting any Xenoestrogens.

I recommend that you only use green tea protein waters the first 3-4 protein waters of the day because for some people green tea may hurt their ability to sleep if they take it within a few hours of bedtime.

By the way, right now you may be thinking that having protein waters all day without any food won't be pleasant. Let me tell you.

With L-Tyrosine and green tea, the 1-Day Diet Plan days *are* pleasant.

You'll notice you'll be able to think more clearly. You'll have more focus. You'll be in a better mood. You'll most likely be more productive. You should also have noticeably more energy as well. Food digestion, especially high carbohydrate food digestion, consumes a massive amount of bodily resources. These resources are freed up on the days you follow the 1-Day Diet Plan.

Note: One reason you get sleepy after a huge meal is your body tries to shut you down and make you sleep. This way, your body can expend far more of its resources to digestion and detoxification than if it also has to keep you awake and moving. Eating a large meal before bedtime, in spite the wives' tales you've been told, is actually healthier and doesn't impact your weight as badly as eating a large meal earlier in the day and continuing to be active.

A great thing about the protein waters is that it only takes a minute to throw in the protein powder and shake it up or stir it. All the time you spent having to make or get food is saved, too. These 7 to 9 protein waters save you time.

Most people think, before doing the 1-Day Diet Plan, that the 7 to 9 protein waters would be a hassle and impractical. But after doing it a few times and getting used to them, then these same people think making or getting food is a big hassle and start to appreciate the convenience of protein waters.

Just please keep an open mind before you even try this.

Once you try the 1-Day Diet Plan and see the immediate results when you wake up the next morning, you'll become a believer. Remember, you can pre-make some or all of the protein waters or green tea protein waters the night before so you don't have to spend any time making them the day you're on the 1-Day Diet Plan. Or make them all in the morning.

Just make sure to have them nearby for when you need to drink them.

Lemons or Lemon Juice

I use lemon juice just because it's easier to deal with than squeezing the juice out of real lemons. But you can use either. Lemon juice has preservatives and isn't as healthy as real lemons. Plus, organic lemons are even better for you. You make the call.

Lemons and lemon juice aid in digestion and they're even more powerful when doing a fast. The 1-Day Diet Plan obviously isn't a traditional fast. But it is similar, just a lot more advanced. Lemon juice and lemons act as a diuretic[18] and help relieve excess bloating.

They're also known to enhance your mood while helping to reduce stress and depression.

Since you're probably not used to not eating for one day, this ability to enhance your mood can't be minimized (just like the other things mentioned in this book in regards to mood enhancers). These mood (and diet) enhancers will help you get through the non-food days since they work on you emotionally and mentally. It won't always be easy, especially the first few times doing the diet. Stack your advantages in order to guarantee your success and commitment to see the diet through.

All in all, lemons or lemon juice are a great addition to the protein waters. Here's how I do it: I pour 1/2 ounce of lemon juice into each protein water.

Just to be clear, I don't measure this out. It's nothing that needs to be exact. Basically, I just pour a little in. Nothing scientific and nothing you need to analyze. Remember, simplicity is the key to following any plan.

The lemon adds a nice taste to the protein waters or green tea protein waters. I especially like lemons with my strawberry flavored protein powder, protein waters.

I buy my lemon juice from the grocery store. I don't remember the exact price, but it's really cheap, around $1.25. Non-organic lemons are around 20 cents each.

I get a 32-ounce bottle of lemon juice and it lasts two to four weeks if you're using the protein waters every other day.

If you get lemons instead, use a lemon for every four protein waters... or about a half lemon for every two protein waters. Just squeeze out the juice into each one equally.

Cinnamon

I love me a little cinnamon!

I like to sprinkle cinnamon into each protein water because cinnamon lowers blood sugar levels,[19] makes you more insulin sensitive,[20] soothes your stomach, and has a positive effect on your brain.[21] The lowering of blood sugar levels and helping with insulin sensitivity are both great for weight loss in general.

The soothing of the stomach and positive effect on how your brain functions are especially ideal for the 1-Day Diet Plan, because your stomach is kind of getting a day off from digestion on the protein water fast days. The cinnamon soothing helps just in case your body doesn't adjust to the diet immediately.

The positive effect on brain function is necessary, again, because it's emotionally and mentally hard for some people not to eat food for a day because it's such an ingrained habit. I recommend you try this out and sprinkle some cinnamon into your protein waters.

No measuring needed. Just sprinkle a little according to your taste preference.

The one thing you should know is that cinnamon doesn't mix well. A lot of it will settle on top. That's fine. Just drink it off the top. Shake it up or stir it in as best you can. But don't worry that it settles on top.

Nicotine Gum

Nicotine gum may be my most controversial suggestion. If it's not for you, then it's not for you. I understand. It's *just* a suggestion and not mandatory to take.

First off, if you are a former smoker, I think you should avoid this tip. If you currently smoke or have never smoked, you should be able to use this tip.

Most people think nicotine is the bad part of cigarettes. And most people would be wrong if they think that. Nicotine is the addictive part of cigarettes. There's a lot of it in there. But the harmful part of cigarettes is all the toxic chemicals added to them and not the nicotine.

To be clear: Cigarettes are bad; nicotine in moderation is good.

What is moderation... about one to two milligrams of nicotine once or twice a day.

Note: There is about 3mg of nicotine in the average cigarette. If the average person smokes a pack of 20 cigarettes a day, that's 60mg of nicotine for the day. That is not moderation.

As you can see, cigarette smokers get way more nicotine compared to what I'm suggesting for you. At one to two milligrams once or twice a day, nicotine gum is *not* addictive. You'll be fine.

If you're a non-smoker, as I have been my entire life, I suspect you will kind of get scared when you hear someone suggestion that you take nicotine. Here's the thing: Nicotine doesn't cause cancer.

Nicotine is actually used in energy drinks in Japan for its positive cognitive effects. Nicotine has cognitive effects just as caffeine does. When both nicotine and caffeine are used in moderation, they combine in a good way for you.

Note: If you get a headache on the first or second day of the 1-Day Diet, it may be due to a withdrawal from caffeine in your diet. To resolve this you can take one caffeine pill in the late morning or early afternoon.

Nicotine has been proven to be a metabolism booster. Ever wonder why a lot of smokers are skinny but then when they stop smoking they gain weight? That's your evidence right there. They are no longer getting nicotine. That results in a slowing down of their metabolisms.

So, how do I suggest you use nicotine?

First, buy a box of nicotine gum that is one to two milligrams in each piece. Do not buy the nicotine gums that have four mg per piece because that's too much nicotine for our purposes.

If you're in the USA, you can get nicotine gum at Walgreens, CVS, or Walmart. If you're not in the USA, I'm not sure where you can get it. But I'm sure nicotine gum is around.

I suggest that you take nicotine gum only if you feel a little "off" while on the protein waters. If this happens, it usually happens in the mid to late afternoon. Pop in a piece of nicotine gum and chew on it for 15-30 minutes. It usually takes about 30 minutes of chewing for the gum to empty out all the nicotine.

Because the nicotine is absorbed through your mouth and into your bloodstream, the mood-enhancing affects are pretty fast. You should feel re-energized and be in a better mood almost immediately.

That's what you want. You want to feel great while on the protein waters.

What I personally found best (and it's different for each person based on all the feedback we've gotten) is to take the three grams of L-Tyrosine in the morning with the first or second protein water and then chew a piece of nicotine gum for 15-30 minutes after the fourth or fifth protein water.

Consider this about nicotine gum: Smokers who are trying to quit smoking are often told to chew 10-24 pieces of nicotine gum a day. As you can see, a single piece of nicotine gum is nowhere near that amount. It is well below a dose that would become addictive. To put things in perspective, nicotine and caffeine are very similar. If you drank a lot of caffeine all the time, you get addicted to it. It is the same thing with nicotine. As I said above, in moderate or low doses, both caffeine and nicotine are actually beneficial to people.

Now, do you have to use nicotine gum? Of course not.

It's just a suggestion that I think would help a lot of people. But it's not necessary if you don't want to use it. The only drawback in my opinion is the cost. Although costs are different, generally speaking, nicotine gum is kind of expensive. 40 pieces of the 2mg nicotine gum at my local drug store cost $15 (as I write this).

Now, for use on the 1-Day Diet Plan protein water days only, 40 pieces last a long time. 40 pieces of gum would last for 40 of the 1-Day Diet Plan days, or 40 protein water fasting days!

Since you can't do the protein waters two days in a row, that means the gum would last at least 80 days if you did the 1-Day Diet Plan every other day which is the maximum rate I ever suggest.

Anyway, the nicotine gum like all these other 1-Day Diet Plan enhancers is just a suggestion and not 100% needed on this plan in order to lose weight. But it does help.

Sometimes, like the first few times you do the plan, nicotine gum can be a huge mental and emotional help for you.

It's worth giving a try. Just keep an open mind.

6
EATING ON NON-DIET DAYS WITH SOME GOTCHAS

Eating on your non-fast days is the easy part!

On the days you are not following the 1-Day Diet Plan, eat pretty much whatever you like. Simple, huh?

Yes. Cheeseburgers, pizza, lasagna, … whatever.

The reason why you can do this is because your body is in nutrient-hoarding mode and not fat-storing mode for one to two days after the 1-Day Diet Plan. In other words, your body is better able to utilize bad foods and digest and discard the nutrients in the bad foods so that they don't get turned into fat or wasted.

Now of course, this isn't giving you permission to eat like a pig. That you *can't* do. Just be sensible and eat your favorite foods in moderation and you'll be fine. But having said that, if you can eat somewhat healthier than the average person on the days you aren't doing the 1-Day Diet Plan, your results will be a little bit better.

What do I suggest you eat on these off days?

I think you should focus on eating eggs (free-range and organic if possible), beans and lentils (both are high in protein and fiber, lentils seems to produce better fat loss than beans), lean grass-fed organic meats, and vegetables (yes, organic when possible).

At very least try to get some of those foods into your eating. (If you're a vegetarian, then obviously eat vegetarian dishes.)

Here is what I want to stress to make things go far more smoothly than they otherwise will if you eat junk. On your off days, if you're going to eat bad foods, eat bad foods at your meals, and not as snacks.

You will naturally begin to snack less the further into your initial month you get. Once you do the 1-Day Diet Plan several times, you'll eventually get away from wanting to eat a lot of snacks. Your body actually starts to teach and show you naturally that a lot of times you're eating snacks, it's because of a habit and not because you're hungry. You will start to notice the difference between being empty and being hungry. It's a subtle, but huge difference.

Note: You may over-eat snacks now, especially sugary and high-starchy carbohydrate based snacks because those become addictive. They provide no nutrition and the more you eat, the more your body craves more of them. The 1-Day Diet begins to reverse this trend quickly.

So, to help the process along faster, I encourage you to eat your bad foods at meals and not between meals. Here is a huge tip for snacking: On the days you're not doing the 1-Day Diet, use the protein waters as snacks between your meals.

Another Thing About Eating What You Want

There are no restrictions on how you eat on your off days, but please try to limit the amount of high calorie, sugar-loaded drinks and alcoholic beverages you have.

Those empty calories don't help the weight loss cause. Don't sabotage your efforts. High sugar liquids are the worst of the worst ways to fight fat. And don't fool yourself into thinking fruit juice is better than Coca-Cola. Unless you use a low-heat blender to juice whole fruit with the fiber and all, then any fruit juice you drink is nothing but a fructose cocktail that will reverse a lot of hard work you do elsewhere.

Note: To reiterate, you can use protein waters between your meals as snacks (and with your meals) as a replacement to high calorie, sugar drinks on the days you're not doing the 1-Day Diet.

Regardless, there are no hardcore restrictions on your free days. If you want to drink sodas with a lot of sugar in them or fruit juices, you can… and you'll still lose weight. *But* you'll lose even more weight if you cut that and some of those bad foods out on your non-protein water days.

The DON'Ts

Fortunately, the list of *don'ts* is small. Here are some things you *can't* do on your 1-Day Diet Plan days.

To get the most weight loss possible, please don't cheat on your protein water. Remember, the 1-Day Diet Plan is just *one* day of dieting. The next day you can go back to eating like normal.

Note: When I say "normal" eating, I mean you can eat your favorite foods in *moderation* and minimize having drinks that have a lot of sugar and calories in them. Don't eat like a pig, at least for the first month on the 1-Day Diet Plan! That's not asking much in order for you to never have to worry about how your body looks ever again.

After the first month on the 1-Day Diet Plan, then if you want to eat a lot of foods, it's more okay. Go ahead. You can always go back to doing the 1-Day Diet Plan to lose any weight you might gain back.

This type of flexibility is why you can't fail on this plan.

After the first month, you are in control of when and how often you'll do the 1-Day Diet Plan. It's not like you'll be doing a strict diet, daily, for weeks or month's non-stop. The beauty of this plan is that you can't even do the diet 2 days in a row even when you're being strict.

For a plan as *simple and effective as The 1-Day Diet Plan* is, make a promise to yourself right now: For each day you're on the 1-Day Diet Plan, give it your full commitment. Remember, tomorrow is a new day and you can go back to eating whatever you want.

Back to the Don'ts

Don't have a protein water fewer than 90 minutes (1.5 hours) after the most recent one. Also, don't drink a protein water more than 150 minutes (2.5 hours) after the most recent one. You need to stay within the 90 to 150 minutes (1.5-2.5 hours) timeframe when spacing out your protein waters.

Don't have less than 9 ounces (250ml) or more than 14 ounces (400ml) of water (or green tea) in each protein water. You need to stay within the 9 to 14 ounces (250 to 400ml) of water range. Based off feedback, this is the ideal range to keep you from feeling bloated since for some people this may seem like a lot of liquids. Anything less than 9 ounces is really not enough water or green tea. I personally use about 10ish ounces.

Don't eat anything on the 1-Day Diet Plan day. This is a modified intermittent fasting day. Eating *anything* on this day ruins some of the diet's effects (but again, if you feel the need to break off the diet and eat dinner, do so). Also, drinking anything *except* water or tea between each protein water would greatly reduce the effectiveness of this diet.

If you follow the outline of the plan, you won't feel starved at all. You may feel empty though. That's normal and expected. If you do feel empty or even hungry (sometimes it can happen), then just drink some plain water until your next protein water.

Usually the time you will feel empty or maybe a little hungry is somewhere around the fourth and fifth protein waters for the day in the afternoon. It usually goes away after the next protein water.

And again, it won't feel like you're starving. The emptiness you feel will help teach and correct your emotional eating habits too.

Why?

This is because you'll soon intuitively see that a lot of times you eat mostly out of habit and not true hunger. After following the 1-Day Diet Plan for a few weeks, most people will develop the natural ability to auto-correct when they eat based off their hunger and not out of habit. A great benefit of this diet is that your body tells you to eat only when you're hungry. It'll do this without you even trying to eat less often.

No coffee

Coffee is a no-no (hard for me to say). If you need the pick-me-up of coffee, use the diet enhancers. Those diet enhancers are proven to work. If you need the coffee flavor, get a coffee-flavored protein powder, like the one I mentioned previously. If you need the caffeine in coffee, use a caffeine pill instead. If you can drink coffee plain, then yes, you can have coffee. The problem is people cheat and add stuff to their coffees and this is where we run into problems. It's just easier to say no coffee.

Again, use the diet enhancers. They make the 1-Day Diet Plan easier to do mentally and they enhance your weight loss results. You don't need to use the diet enhancers on the days you're not on the 1-Day Diet Plan.

You can't drink any calorie drinks on the 1-Day Diet Plan days.

The only thing you can have besides the protein waters is plain water or tea between each protein water.

Most people don't even feel the need to drink water between each protein water. You'll get plenty of water in each protein water.

Another don't: Don't chew gum with sugar in it. You can chew sugar-free gum between protein waters, but I even advise against that. If you must chew gum, I recommend you chew nicotine gum (except ex-smokers) as part of the diet enhancers. Use the 1-2mg pieces of nicotine gum. They are safe and non-addictive. Chew the nicotine gum for 15-30 minutes between protein waters when you feel the need.

> **Note:** Use the nicotine gum no more than twice a day (once in the morning and once in the afternoon).

More Don'ts

Don't have fewer than seven protein waters in a day and don't have more than nine in a day.

It's your decision on how many protein waters to have each day as long as it's from 7 to 9 protein waters each day. People are different. The best results seem to come from having 9 a day. But for some people, it may be impractical to fit in that many.

For me personally, I usually have 9 protein waters and space them out 90-105 minutes apart. But sometimes I'm a little busier than normal and 9 protein waters are just too hard to fit in and remember… even when I pre-make them early in the morning and use a timer.

On my busy days, I sometimes have just 7 protein waters and space them out 2 hours to 2 hours and 15 minute apart. Figure out what works for you. Just stay within the guidelines.

There's a lot of flexibility built into this plan so that you won't feel like it is one size fits all.

Just use your good judgment and follow the outline and rules and you'll be fine.

Don't use fewer than 10 grams of protein and don't use more than 20 grams of protein in each protein water. For most protein waters, I personally use just 10 grams of protein in the scoop. Each protein powder is different, so you'll have to calculate out how much 10 grams of actual protein is. Not all of the scoops in protein powders are the same size and not all the grams in protein powder are protein. There are carbs, fat, and additive grams in there too.

But 10 grams of protein is all you need, usually. However, you can use more than 10 grams of protein if you feel you need it. If you notice some hunger issues, bump it up to 15 grams of protein in protein waters.

From all the feedback we've gotten, people have lost a lot of weight using 20 grams of protein in each protein water. (If you're a man reading this, instead of using 10-15 grams of protein per protein water, I advise you to use 15-20 grams of protein per protein water.)

In my opinion, using 20 grams in each protein water is a waste of protein powder for most women. It's simply not needed. The only times you should even consider using more than 10 grams of protein in a protein water is if you felt empty prior to the protein water. In that case, you can bump up the 10 grams of protein to 15-20 grams for your next protein water.

If you were to do that, you'll most likely only need to use that amount once or twice a day.

So to be clear: Use 10 grams of protein in each protein water. But you can boost it up to 15 to 20 grams of protein for one to two or even more protein waters for the day. If after a day doing the 1-Day Diet with 10 grams of protein per protein water doesn't feel right to you, then the next protein water day boost that up to 15 grams of protein per protein water for *all* protein waters. It's your call. You know your body and how you're feeling on these protein waters better than me or anyone else. Use the built-in flexibility designed into this diet to your fullest advantage.

7
1-DAY DIET PLAN Q&A'S

Q: Can you use the 1-Day Diet Plan with other diets?

A: Yes and no. On the actual days of doing the 1-Day Diet Plan, you have to do it as outlined. So in that regard, no, you can't do other diets. But on the days you're not doing the 1-Day Diet Plan, yes, you can follow another diet if you want (within reason).

Still, my suggestion is to simply eat like "normal," but just try to eat a little bit healthier on the off-days.

Q: Do I have to exercise?

A: No.

But in the next section I'll talk about how exercise can enhance your weight loss results. And no, you don't need to go crazy with exercise. Just a little bit of exercise strategically used will accelerate your weight loss a lot.

Q: Can I eat cheeseburgers, pizzas, and other "bad" foods on my off-days?

A: Yes but… *Please* be reasonable. Don't eat like a pig. Eat them in moderation.

One of the reasons why this diet is so easy and successful is because you won't feel deprived for days, weeks, or months at a time like on a typical diet. Unlike most diets where you feel deprived of your favorite foods for weeks (or months) non-stop, with this diet, you know it's only one day you have to be strict.

The next day you can go back to eating your favorite foods, within reason.

This is a very powerful concept because it empowers you to be able to do this type of dieting for the rest of your life. Another thing in regards to eating bad foods... you have a one to two hour "window of opportunity" right after exercising where your body goes into a hyper state of nutrient hording due to the need for nutrients immediately caused from the exercising. This is the best time to eat bad foods and not worry about them going to your waist. Remember that!

Q: Can I do the 1-Day Diet for two or more days in a row?

A: *Nooooo!* Don't do that, ever!

Non-consecutive days is the ideal way to use this form of dieting for the best weight loss results. This dieting strategy has been thoroughly tested and used by a lot of people (including professional athletes). The testing showed that two or more days in a row is *not* as effective as following the 1-Day Diet Plan on non-consecutive days.

You will actually lose *less* weight if you were to do two or more days in a row of the 1-Day Diet Plan. Plus doing it two or more days in a row is mentally and emotionally difficult. We're trying to get away from difficulties so you can easily follow a diet that's easy, cheap, and amazingly effective. It's critical that you don't feel as though you're suffering.

So please stick to the plan.

Q: What is the best way to time each protein water so you don't miss one or mess up the timing?

A: The best way to do this is to use your cell phone alarm. Immediately after you finish a protein water, set your cell phone alarm for around two hours later, or however long you want to set between the protein waters (within the guidelines).

Then when it rings, get your protein water and drink it. Repeat that each time.

Q: Does this diet work for vegetarians?

A: Yep. Simply eat whatever you normally eat on the day you're not on the 1-Day Diet Plan.

Q: Can I use soy protein instead of whey?

A: *No!* Absolutely not. Soy products, including soy protein[22], are generally bad for you. Don't believe the health food gurus: soy products are unhealthy.

Without going into a long-winded explanation, to put it simply, soy messes up your thyroid and causes your hormones to become unbalanced. Soy basically causes your thyroid to become more and more under-active (hypothyroidism) over time.

Although soy is bad for men, women, and children, it's especially bad for men and boys because soy is an estrogen-mimic. In essence, it will feminize little boys and men by altering their hormones and creating an environment within the body where it's estrogen-dominant instead of testosterone-dominant.

> **Note:** Real soy sauce is safe because the soy has been fermented[23] and it promotes none of the negative side effects that other types of soy produce.

Q: Can I use milk in the protein waters?

A: No. Protein waters are *not* protein shakes. There's a good reason why they're called protein *waters*. These protein waters aren't meant to be meal replacements and they're not meant to be loaded with extra calories.

Also, homogenized and pasteurized milk is unhealthy and bad for weight loss. So when you and your family ever *do* drink milk, find a local producer who sells whole, raw milk. If you or your family are lactose intolerant, you will find that malady non-existent if you drink only delicious, whole raw milk (or goat milk).

Q: How fast do I drink the protein waters?

A: Drink them as fast as possible and as fast as you're comfortable with. Basically, that means drink each one in about 5 minutes or less.

Q: I don't like the taste of protein waters. Is there anything I can do to improve the taste?

A: Yes, sprinkle in Stevia. Just a little. And remember the cinnamon boost too. Don't sprinkle in anything else. Protein waters won't taste as good as protein shakes. Accept that. But you can make protein waters taste better with Stevia and/or cinnamon. Also, you can add extra protein to each protein water (up to 20 grams of protein) to improve the taste.

Q: Is there anything else I can use in the protein waters to improve the taste or help fill me up so I'm not as hungry between each one?

A: Yes. You can use sugar free Metamucil (or a generic equivalent). Each teaspoon of Metamucil contains about three grams of fiber in it. You can use this with every protein water, every other one, or however you want. The orange flavored Metamucil tastes especially good with chocolate protein powders (in my opinion). It adds a nice rich texture to each protein water and helps to control your hunger. I personally use Walmart's Equate Fiber Therapy brand, which is basically identical to Metamucil. It costs about $9 for 2 pounds and 180 doses. This will last you months, even if you use it a lot in your protein waters.

8
HOW EXERCISE FITS INTO THE 1-DAY DIET PLAN

To be clear, you *don't* need to exercise while doing the 1-Day Diet Plan. Still, exercise will enhance your weight loss results and allow you to lose more weight, faster. You should develop and keep more lean muscle mass when you exercise. This increases your body's metabolism and thus helps increase the rate of fat loss.

But exercise isn't required for the 1-Day Diet Plan to work. Don't get hung up on having to exercise. If you're really ambitious and want to lose as much weight as possible, as fast as possible, then include exercise into this program. If you're kind of lazy or too busy to fit in exercise, then don't stress about it.

Can you still lose 20 or more pounds in a month without exercise while doing the 1-Day Diet Plan three times a week or every other day for a month? A resounding *yes* is the answer. I do encourage you to add exercise to this program because I want you to get the best results possible, as fast as possible.

I want you to have a total health plan and not just a diet plan. So in this section, I'm going to share with you how to enhance your 1-Day Diet Plan weight loss results by including some exercise.

What we've found is the best weight loss results from exercise while doing the 1-Day Diet Plan program is to exercise the day *after* you do the 1-Day Diet Plan protein waters.

Why is that? It's because the body is more insulin sensitive and extra sensitive to burning fat the day after the 1-Day Diet Plan. It doesn't really matter what exercise you do. The key is that you sweat while exercising. Your body is in an amplified fat-burning mode so take advantage of it and do some exercise.

Planning Exercise

Let's map this out.

If you were to do the 1-Day Diet Plan every other day for a month; that means you'll follow the program for 15 days out of the month. On those other 15 days, simply do some sort of exercise that causes you to get a good sweat, even if it takes only 5 minutes of your time.

That's it.

If you can work up a sweat by doing a little bit of exercise every one of those 30 days during the first month you're doing the 1-Day Diet Plan, that'll get you some incredible results.

And you don't have to work out for one hour. If you can work up a sweat in 5-10 minutes, that's all you need. Maybe do something such as vacuuming your home if that's enough to make you sweat a little.

Now, if you do the 1-Day Diet Plan twice a week (we suggest Mondays and Thursdays), then you should work out on Tuesdays and Fridays. This isn't to say you can't exercise on other days. We've found that the next best day to use exercise to burn off more fat while doing the 1-Day Diet Plan is to exercise the day you're doing the 1-Day Diet Plan. This gets great results also.

Now, if you do the 1-Day Diet Plan once a week or whenever you feel like it, the best way to include exercise is to do it the day of the 1-Day Diet Plan AND the day after it.

I encourage you to add exercise to this program to maximize your weight loss. You don't need a complicated exercise program. The main thing with exercise while on this program is to work up a good sweat doing whatever you want. If that means walking, then walk.

That's really all the exercise you'll need while on this diet. Again, just to be clear: You *don't* need to exercise at all if you don't want to or you can't. You'll still lose a lot of weight without doing any type of exercise.

If you want a more complete exercise plan, I suggest you read my book, *Running Sucks!*[1]

9
RECAP

A recap would help tie up loose ends you may have.

The 1-Day Diet Plan requires you to drink 7 to 9 protein waters spaced out every 1.5 to 2.5 hours apart (that means about every 90 to 150 minutes).

Each protein water will contain 10 to 15 grams of protein and you'll need 9 to 14 ounces of water for each one. Drink each one in 5 minutes or less. As fast as you're comfortable drinking them. Then once you're done drinking one, set your cell phone alarm to ring for the next protein water.

For the best and fastest weight loss results, do the 1-Day Diet Plan every other day for the first month.

The very first time you do the 1-Day Diet Plan, you will most likely lose 2 to 5 pounds. After that, you'll most likely lose a pound or two each time you follow the plan for the first month. After you've completed the first month, you'll know how powerful this is as a diet. At times you may lose water weight and then regain it back. This is normal and nothing to worry about. Think of it like two to three steps forward and one step back. Sometimes it will be one step forward and one step back. This is nothing to be concerned about. Continue on with the diet.

With the knowledge that this diet works, after the first month it's up to you how often you'll do the 1-Day Diet Plan in order to lose weight, maintain your weight, and or do it for the healthy cleansing and detoxification effects.

I personally do it once a week for the health benefits and to stay near my ideal weight. But some people have stopped using the 1-Day Diet Plan for weeks and months. Whenever they're not happy with their weight, they simply jump back into doing the 1-Day Diet Plan a few times to lose the necessary weight and then go back to their normal eating.

Consider the periodic 1-Day Diet Plan days as your insurance policy against you ever getting fat again (once you've lost all the weight you need to lose).

Like most of the truly great things in life, this is simple. Nothing complicated. Simple is easy to stick with. If you do it, you'll lose more weight than you ever thought possible, quickly and easily.

Please don't be that person who comes up with excuses or criticisms without even trying this out. If you don't think this will work, ok fine, try it anyway and prove to yourself that it doesn't work. Keep an open mind. This is truly a breakthrough diet whether you realize it or not. Suspend your judgment and simply do the diet.

Our results

After a few days you'll see the fast results. Those fast results will give you the encouragement that this diet does in fact work and you'll continue doing it.

It's as simple as that.

You don't have to wait weeks or months to see results. After a few days you'll know whether or not it's working for you. Remember, professional athletes (both women and men) rely on this diet strategy. It would be dumb for them to trust it if it wasn't proven because it could cost them millions of dollars by not giving them the best body possible to perform at the highest level possible.

So, if they can trust this diet with that much at stake, you can at least trust it enough to give it an honest try a few times to see what all the hype is about.

This is your time to shine. Make it happen. Peel off your fat and show the world the *new You!*

Section 2:

The 5:2 Diet Cheat Sheet: Breakthrough 2-Days-a-Week Dieting

10
INTRODUCING THE 5:2 DIET CHEAT SHEET

No doubt you've heard about this thing called *The 5:2 Diet*. You may have seen all the books, articles, cookbooks, web sites, and so on. So why do you need yet *another* book about it?

For one thing, this gives you the details you need most and eliminates all the extra things that don't matter at all. Let's face it – you want to know what the 5:2 Diet is all about, you want to know how to do it, why it works, and then you want to move on down the road and begin losing weight.

Also, I have considerably more experience with Intermittent Fasting than the people who have written about the 5:2 Diet in the last few months. I've been doing or writing about Intermittent Fasting since 2009. With that, I add in some of my own secrets to make the 5:2 Diet even better.

I don't believe in wasting your time. I strive to give my readers the Stuff and never the Fluff.

As you may know, I have written extensively about the popular diets out there. I want you to be healthy and have the body you want, not waste your time, waste your money, or waste your waist!

Enough people asked about the 5:2 Diet to cause me to research heavily what it was all about, follow it for a few months for my first-hand account. It was then critical to take the time to write a book about it so that you, my readers, got a chance to learn about this thing without spending too much time or money. You can learn the basics very quickly.

On top of that, the 5:2 Diet is a nice complement to the 1-Day Diet. You're actually getting a second diet in this 1-Day Diet book.

Why This Cheat Sheet?

You will soon learn all about the 5:2 Diet in this "cheat sheet," a guide that short-circuits your way to understanding what it's all about. The 5:2 Diet is not just a diet. As a matter of fact, one of the most important elements of the 5:2 Diet is this:

When you eat is far more important than *what* you eat!

It's true. You actually will eat just about anything and everything you want on the 5:2 Diet. That makes it amazing. And while I see massive evidence that a natural, organic, low-carbohydrate eating regimen is healthier than most if not all alternatives, there is a major aspect of the 5:2 Diet that improves health benefits even if you eat a lot of carbs; and of course you should lose weight too.

Here you learn:

- The 5:2 Diet's health benefits
- The 5:2 Diet's weight loss benefits
- The 5:2 Diet's feel-good factor

It's that third benefit I like about it. Although I am in good shape, and was before I researched the 5:2 Diet for you, I followed the 5:2 Diet for some time as I was studying its benefits and problems. I found that I never had the sluggish feeling that I've had when trying other eating plans in the past.

Note: To be fair, I am so used to returning to my 1-Day Diet: the Fastest "Diet" in the World, and while it's sort of the 5:2 Diet on the proverbial super-powerful steroids, that may be why when I switched full-time to the 5:2 Diet for a few weeks it was no trouble for me. I doubt it will be much trouble for you either, especially if you've been trying the previous 1-Day Diet section of this book. Still, the first few days on the 5:2 Diet, you may feel some discomfort while you tackle the 5:2 Diet but that should even out after a couple of weeks.

As I said, the 1-Day Diet is like the 5:2 Diet on steroids (not that I suggest steroids). One of the reasons the 5:2 Diet ever hit my radar is that I'd heard how my 1-Day Diet told had some similarities to the 5:2 Diet. The 5:2 Diet is a great follow-up *or* ramp-up for starting my powerful 1-Day Diet.

Okay... Place your seats in their upright position and strap yourself in. We're about to dive right into the 5:2 Diet!

The 5:2 Diet Explained in Just One Sentence!

As with just about any diet, the fundamentals of the 5:2 Diet are simple and quick to explain. But it's the details that make it successful; otherwise this book would be about one sentence long.

For example, if I were going to tell you what a low-carb diet is all about in a single sentence, I'd say:

"Increase your fats and proteins and eliminate all starchy carbs."

And yet there are so many details about a low-carb diet that separate the success from the failures that the single sentence description, if anything, does more harm than good.

I want you to agree that you need to understand some fundamentals about the 5:2 Diet before it can possibly work for you. At the same time I want to make things as clear as quickly as I can. So I'm going to begin with a one-sentence description of the 5:2 Diet and although it's not *nearly* enough for you to be successful on the 5:2 Diet, it does give us a platform to work from for the rest of the book:

"Eat what you want to eat 5 days each week and fast on the other 2 days."

Wow. If you really knew nothing about the 5:2 Diet before this, that one-sentence description may make you hesitate.

Who wants to go two days a week without eating anything?

The answer is: Nobody. That's just why the details behind the 5:2 Diet are so critical. Now that you know the very foundation of the 5:2 Diet you'll learn from the details we cover in the rest of this section that you *can* follow the 5:2 Diet without nearly the angst you may have considered from reading its one-sentence description.

So come with me and I'll give you the nitty gritty. You can do this. It's *much* easier than it sounds.

11
MAKING THE 5:2 DIET'S "2" MUCH BETTER

From the 1-Day Diet, you already know that fasts, especially *intermittent fasts,* are not impossible or even difficult to follow. Also, a fast doesn't have to be a 100% *complete fast* to be effective. Remember, you can gain health benefits and weight loss benefits from a partial fast.

Note: The Oregon Institute of Science and Medicine has been on the forefront of fasting research for the last several years[25]. You can learn additional information about the scientific background of fasting from their articles.

Fasting also, as I said earlier, ramps up weight loss. People who fast tend to lose weight. This is also true if over the same period of time, the people eat exactly the same number of calories and the same amount of food... but fast here and there. There's something about the periods of fasting, which seem to kick weight-loss into high gear. It's a combination of factors and almost certainly has some to do with our bodies utilizing fat stores.

One reason it is so easy to gain weight in such a short period of time is because our body will send excess energy to fat cells, increasing their size. This is stored energy for later use in case we go without nourishment for a period of time unexpectedly. The fasting therefore utilizes that stored energy that we know as fat.

Note: Several theories have been thrown out there as to why fasting triggers the reactions it does in our bodies. I have a suspicion that we were created this way in order to be able to live through long periods of near or total starvation, as is sometimes the case with prisoners of war, people lost in the desert or arctic regions, and so on. If missing our regular meals over an extended period immediately caused us to be unable to do much of anything, then we would be more likely to die in those situations.

But as you know, if you've ever heard of those kinds of stories, people have lived an extremely long time on very little nourishment. The enzymes and our bodies work together in starvation mode, possibly by shutting down some of the less important resources in our body, in order to actually strengthen some of the energy and life-sustaining functions during periods of starvation.

Performing an I.F. the 5:2 Way

Let's say that you do an intermittent fasting program where you skip breakfast every day and eat only between the hours of 12 noon and 8 PM at night. The amount that you eat is exactly the same as the amount that you eat when you do not do the fast. It turns out, you will lose weight and obtain almost every benefit of fasting that you would obtain from fasting straight through for two or three days at a time and then eating normally. In other words, if the number of hours that you fast each day totals two or three days of fasting over a week, the benefits of the more concentrated fasting appears to go to both kinds of fasters – those who fasted all at once, and those who perform the fast over a period of several days!

Now that opens up all sorts of interesting possibilities, doesn't it? Those of us who avoid fasting like the plague because who wants to go a day or more without eating, now have a very high probability of success with fasting. All of us can go a *short* time without eating even if we normally would be eating during that time on other days. In addition, all of us can eat less one or two days a week. This *reduced consumption fast* never leaves us starving because we do eat during the "fasting" time periods; we just eat *less*.

The 2 in the 5:2

It is that last sentence that enables almost everybody to have success with the 5:2 Diet. Because here is exactly what the *2* in the 5:2 Diet is all about:

Our 5:2 Diet's fast is a modified fast as well as an intermittent fast because we only do it two non-consecutive days a week. For example, when on the 5:2 Diet, I fast each Monday and Thursday. (The actual days you pick don't matter, just be sure they are not next to each other consecutively. A day or two or three days between each fasting day is best to help ensure that you stick with the plan.)

On the two fasting days, you will eat only 25% of your normal amount of food.

The rest of the week, you eat whatever you want as if you were not doing anything special the other two days!

Why 5:2's Success

It is my suspicion that you are already curious as to how well you can do on the 5:2 Diet. Now that you know more about it, and what you know about it now is the "punch-line" of the diet - by that I mean, those two days when you eat 25% of your normal amount of food are really the only times you do anything special.

None of us want to go two days without food each week, but couldn't all of us go two days a week with a *reduced* amount of food?

A Numerical Example

Assume you're female and normally try to eat 2,200 calories each day on regular, non-fasting days. This means that on fasting days you can eat a total of only 550 calories. This limits the calories you can have at each of 3 meals to 184 calories.

184 calories is not much. How on earth can you live on 184 calories per meal?

You cannot. Fortunately you don't have to. Remember that's not the goal. The goal is to only do that twice a week, and although a complete fast would otherwise boost your weight loss (not necessarily fat loss) tremendously, complete fasting on those two days could be a difficult task to maintain. When difficulty is introduced into any eating plan, the success rate of that eating plan is dramatically reduced. Simple and easy is best and the 5:2 Diet is both simple and easy.

Can I Be Direct?

Can I be very direct and stern with you for a moment?

You must do something different in order to lose weight from what you're doing now. If you do nothing, you will see no change. If you didn't need to lose weight, or didn't want to help someone who needs to lose weight, then you wouldn't have gotten this book. You bought this book knowing that there would have to be a change and that you would not be making every meal a big bowl of ice cream.

For those who read the term "fasting" and began shutting down, *you* are the reason for my being stern. Unless you have a magic genie in a bottle, you must change something to lose weight. And the 5:2 Diet approach to fasting is a superb way... especially when combined with the 1-Day Diet.

This directness is not needed for everyone who gets this book. Most people understand there has to be change. Most people understand that they are going to notice that change. Otherwise, if losing weight required absolutely no effort or no noticeable change, everyone would be slim and trim.

I wasn't going to not include the small section about change because of two factors:

1. I never want to imply that fasting days are difficult.
2. Some people who begin the 5:2 Diet complain that they don't think the fasting days are easy enough to follow. If you happen to be one of those people, I needed to be somewhat stern and say "you've got to do something! Why not just try this for three weeks?" I'm trying to help you so please don't take my being stern personally.

Having said that... if you happen to be one of these people, I want to follow-up with some excellent news. There are many ways to adapt the 5:2 Diet plan to make it far easier.

That's what the next section is all about.

Variations on the 2

The 5:2 Diet is extremely flexible. Always be honest and accurate about the amount of food that you eat. The best way to ensure that you eat only 25% or less calories on your fast days is to measure your food and monitor the calories accurately. Plus, you could eat all of your food on your fasting days in one "large meal," two smaller meals, or three very small meals (more on this later).

Some people will do better eating three smaller meals so they do not get extremely hungry on fasting days. Other people have no problem waiting until, say, dinner in order to eat one large meal on fasting day and go to bed feeling extremely satisfied.

Some people find that a green smoothie drink works well for one of their fasting day meals. As long as you use little or no fruit, and I would suggest sweetening your green smoothie with Stevia[26] and eliminating all of the fruit completely from the smoothie, you could make a vegetable smoothie that's extremely low calorie and yet produces nice enzymes for your body to utilize until your next meal.

Some protein powder in that green smoothie (again, check the calories, because you must be highly accurate and honest that you are only getting 25% of your normal caloric intake) gives you even more long-term energy out of that green smoothie. The vegetables will give you immediate energy, and the proteins will give you longer-term energy, so you truly have very little hunger during the hours between your smoothie and your next meal.

The Problem with Fruits

Fruits are tricky.

I realize many of you love fruits, so do I, but the fructose inside fruits is dangerously high given the rest of the typical Western diet. So many fruits are often eaten without any skins. Think of orange juice sold in cartons and people who use juicers to drink only the juice of fruits and not the pulp or skin. In addition, today's fruits are mostly grown on non-organic farms and the pesticides inside them can easily fight any nutrients that might be in the fruit.

To keep your fasting days from getting out of hand, and to be able to eat a reasonable amount of food, you already know that you should avoid all desserts on those days. I strongly suggest that you avoid all fruit as well. If you must have some fruit, eat a few berries and if you mix them such as blueberries, strawberries, and blackberries it's even better. A mix helps ensure you get good nutrients from the fruit but that you don't overdo the caloric impact (more accurately, the glycemic index's impact) from the fruit that you eat.

We'll talk more about the non-fasting days of the 5:2 Diet in the next chapter, but it should be obvious to you that only five days where you can eat anything you want, the more you overdo and indulge the slower your weight loss is going to be, and the slower the healthy effects of the 5:2 Diet will show themselves.

If possible, if you get a sweet tooth during this diet, even on your non-fasting days, do your best to grab some berries as I've described here. Use the berries to help bypass that sweet tooth craving. Even the berries are high in sugar with their fructose, but they have much less impact on your thighs and hips than other kinds of fruit in general.

The 5:2 Diet is Flexible in More Ways Too

We will talk more about other variations that may suit you better when going on the 5:2 Diet. I want you to have success with this and not give up. Keeping the 5:2 Diet simple and designed based on your personal preferences, will help ensure that you stick with it and enjoy the whole process.

> **Note:** As you can see, fasting doesn't have to be torture! Quite the opposite. If it were difficult, I would never suggest it or have written this book. Difficult diets don't work for me, they don't work for you, and they don't work for anybody.

All About the 5:2 Diet's "5"-Based Food

As I described in the previous chapter, the 5:2 Diet is extremely flexible.

In addition to adjusting the ways that you perform the fast, you truly can eat whatever you want to eat on the days that you don't fast. Remember though, to the extent that you don't overdo starchy carbs and desserts; to that extent you will lose weight faster than if you ate all of that stuff on non-fasting days.

This is not a cop out. I stand by what I said - you can eat whatever you want on the non-fasting days.

You May Not Want to Over-Indulge

Fortunately, most people who have tried this diet, including myself, don't *want* to binge on non-fasting days. You simply don't wake up starving after a fast day. I don't feel the need to run to the nearest grocery store for ice cream or cheesecake!

I awake feeling pretty good after a day of fasting on 25% of my regular consumption. And it is that feel-good feeling that I believe encourages me not to go overboard for the rest of that day. I know that I can eat all the food I want, and with that freedom, I often don't want to binge in any way. I also find that I want to limit my sweets. To be truthful, I don't even want sweets after the first week on the 5:2 Diet. That's great news because the more sweets that we eat the more we crave them. It's a bad roller coaster ride.

We Need to Talk About What You Eat

I simply cannot continue on until I give you a short introduction to the world of food today. The bottom line is: the food that almost everybody eats today, in Western civilization, is horrible. Much of the problem is from the FDA (*Food and Drug Administration*) and the USDA (United States Department of Agriculture) when they tell us what is healthy and what is not.[27]

Doesn't it seem as though people are fatter, sicker, and physically more decrepit than they were 30+ years ago? Our waist sizes have radically changed in the last 30 years.

Looking around, I'm sure you understand this. There is a problem that your body will attempt to cling to fat if you have many toxins in your system. Your body will fight weight loss until you are able to eat good foods which not only removes toxins, but which also don't replace the old toxins that are removed.

Where do we get many of our toxins today? We get them from the foods that we eat. The very food that we eat is toxic including some food we formerly thought was healthy including a lot of grains and fruit. Pesticides in foods are toxins, but even organic grains and fruit in large quantities harm our bodies and reduce our bodies' ability to throw off toxins.

A Warning is in Order – Fruit-Based Dangers

I want to return to a subject I touched on earlier. That subject is fruit.

Fruit in *moderation* is great. Fruit contains antioxidants and eating a variety of fruit of various colors throughout the week, with an extra emphasis on low-glycemic berries over higher-impact sugary fruits such as oranges and bananas, gives you nutrition your body needs.

But when it comes to fruit, many health writers have led you astray. Fruit today is often promoted as a healthy replacement for the calories and other nutrients that you would get from animal proteins and fats from nuts and oils.

Eating fruit the way it comes off the tree or vine (and organically grown) is a fantastic way to get some nutrients that your body loves (in moderation)! Eating dried fruit (sold in schools now instead of candy bars) removes the water, which makes you feel full and leaves you wanting more. That's not good. Fruit juice is hardly better than full-calorie soda;[28] tons of fructose sugar without any of the fiber to slow down the sugar's toxic effects.

> **Note:** Both diet *and* regular sodas contain a preservative called *benzoate*[29] to help maintain freshness. Benzoate interacts with your body's Vitamin C and breaks down to benzene, which is suspected to be a carcinogen.

I want you to begin limiting your intake of fruit not just on the 5:2 Diet, but even if you quit the 5:2 Diet and go on a different diet or a different lifestyle or no diet whatsoever. I want you to begin questioning the amount of fruit that you really should eat. For the most part, fruit is a sugar that your body gets way too much of.

Also, high fructose corn syrup is in virtually every packaged product sold in a grocery store. Our bodies were never designed to have high quantities of fructose.

But What About Fruit's Fiber?

How much fiber is enough?

Fiber is vital to keep food flowing through your body the way it should. It's been said that one needs from 35 to 50 grams of fiber daily to stay regular. This is a general rule of thumb, but there is one even better.

If you are honest with yourself that you truly have healthy, good stools on a regular basis, you almost certainly get enough fiber. Your gut will react to too much or too little and you'll be the first to know if something is askew if you are not getting a proper amount, either on the high side or the low side.

Long-term bowel movement problems indicate a sure sign that you need to address your gut.

Probiotics, fermented food, and more fiber is almost always the trio in short supply when gut problems are present. Still, too much fiber can cause loose stools. If you've been supplementing with fiber or eating fruit for fiber and you haven't seen good results, stop the supplementation and fruit and try to maintain a good level of fibrous veggies, seeds, and nuts for a week or two to see if anything changes. If not, you certainly should see a physician to make sure there is nothing else going on that should be addressed medically.

About Processed Foods

Processed food isn't food. No book about dieting, food, and health would be complete if you didn't understand something incredible. A study recently published in the *Journal of Applied Toxicology*[30] showed that thousands of consumer products – processed "foods" – contains hormone-mimicking preservatives.

That literally means, you are getting hormone therapy every time you eat a box of <*fill-in-favorite-junk-food-here*>.

And guess what? If you don't need hormone therapy, you shouldn't have it!

The primary and most dangerous health culprit in processed food is the *paraben* which is often found in processed food preservatives at a rate of *one million times higher than estrogen levels found in human breasts*. These parabens mimic estrogen hormones. And the parabens are found in food, drugs, and cosmetics.

The reason women tend to have more fat than men is because women have over 1,000 times the concentration of estrogen receptors that men have. Our world constantly floods our bodies with estrogen and parabens that mimic estrogen. If you're a woman and are afraid of excess estrogens in your body, consider what it does to your husband or boyfriend who were designed to have far less estrogen levels than you. And more frightening, consider what the environment's excess estrogen does to your children!

A wide range of Erectile Dysfunction drugs are sold now for men. A vast number of breast cancers are found in both women *and* men. Children are reaching puberty at ages as young as eight years old. Hormones are powerful and can be good or bad depending on their quantities. Estrogen is an especially insidious hormone these days given how rampant it is in the environment... in preservatives, in cosmetics, in drugs, and in soy.

If knowing this keeps you from picking up the next box of <*fill-in-your-favorite-food-here*> the next time you go grocery shopping and forces you to run instead to your organic produce section, then I've done my job.

Note: By the way, good food, real food, food that is good for your body, is not boring or bland food. Those who understand how to eat well also understand the importance of spices. Spices are the underutilized secret of good food *and nutrition*. There's a reason why history books are filled with centuries of explorers and pirates hunting for the best spice routes in the medieval world. Spices make food taste good and pack a powerful nutritional punch.

The Problem with Fats is that Fat is a Solution

Probably many people have worked hard to convince you that fat in your diet needs to be reduced and replaced with grains and fruit. For 30 or 40 years now the government's Food Pyramid put fat at the very apex of the pyramid, the smallest part of the graphic, to warn you against the dangers of fat.

Gary Taubes of the Nutrition Science Initiative[31] wrote an outstanding, but extremely high-level, advanced, scientific volume entitled, "Good Calories, Bad Calories" in which he shows systematically how adding fat back into your diet will systematically force your cells to release fat stores and you'll lose weight. The recommendations that led to the government's Food Pyramid said animal fat is bad for us and we should not eat meat.

Problems exist with this view. Having said that, certainly not all fats are good for you. But certainly a lot of grains and even a lot of fruit aren't necessarily good for you either.

Good Fat is Good for You

To begin getting your weight loss (and overall health) into gear, you need to eat more fat. Fat should provide at least 35% of your diet with most of the fat coming from animal sources such as grass-fed beef, wild Alaskan salmon (which has low levels of mercury unlike just about any other fish),[32] farm-raised nitrate-free nitrite-free pork (if you eat pork), free-range chickens, organic seeds, nuts, and healthy oils.

So fats are good? Yes, but not all of them! There is a huge difference between manufactured fats and naturally occurring healthy fats.

Both the health and food experts such as Gary Taubes *and* the traditional FDA-like proponents and medical schools agree that trans fats are bad for us. Trans fats can be a type of *unsaturated fats*.[33] Stay away from any kind of fat or cooking oil labeled trans fat, unsaturated fat, monounsaturated fat, or polyunsaturated fat. This deadly fat messes up your whole body, from your hormones to your heart to your cholesterol.

Polyunsaturated vegetable oils and fats can become toxic and unstable when heated due to creation of free radicals that damage our cells. Trans fats from hydrogenated oils and margarine are like plastics. They interfere with cells communications between each other, which leads to health dysfunction and chaos at the cell level.

Many fats are great though. Tropical fats are wonderful for us.[34] Cook your family's eggs each morning in organic extra virgin coconut oil. Olive oil is also awesome. Make sure you get dark olive oil and always get it in dark, glass bottles because olive oil begins to turn rancid quickly from light. In addition, the lighter-shades of olive oil are indicators of being bleached in peroxide and other solvents and why would you ever want that?

Note: Try organic macadamia nut oil for a nice surprising taste. Ghee is also a wonderful butter.

Speaking of macadamia nuts, organic nuts and seeds are wonderful sources of fats and minerals and vitamins. Make organic nuts and seeds a regular part of your family's diet with a couple of tablespoons of mixed nuts and seeds daily. Did you know that four Brazil nuts each day is all you need to give your body its needed and important selenium?

You know all about margarine, right? Now forget everything you know about it. Margarine is a trans fat. Throw it away *now*. Never use it again.

Buy only organic grass-fed butter. Better yet, you can make your own butter from fresh, raw, whole milk (which you can source at the Weston A Price Institute's web site[35]) for raw, whole milk in the states where it's legal to buy it) and make your own butter. You don't need to keep real butter in your fridge by the way. It stays soft outside the fridge.

Avocados are high in good fat. They provide one of the best sources of fat you can find. Eating a half avocado at lunch and at dinner goes a long way toward fulfilling your hormonal need for good fats.

In summary, a lack of natural fats in your diet makes you gain weight. Healthy fats are *essential* for your cells to work properly to eliminate waste and toxins at your cell level, and freeing up your body to lose weight. Fats stabilize blood sugar levels, decrease cravings, and make you feel full.

Not All Calories are Equal – *Especially* on the 5:2 Diet

A calorie is not a calorie is not a calorie. More accurately, not all calories affect our bodies in the same way.

Most calories from starchy carbohydrates such as grains, corn, and potatoes, impact your weight far more than the same number of calories which come from healthy fat-based foods and calories from protein-based foods such as grass fed beef.

Note: I am not a fan of calorie-counting diets.[36] When someone tries to lose weight solely by eating less, they set themselves up for failure. Our bodies were not designed to live over a long period of time on reduced calorie diets. Yes, the 5:2 Diet does reduce your calories on fasting days. But your body does not go into a starvation mode when you only perform a partial fast and then only do that twice a week. Statistically, every person who has ever gone on a severe calorie restricted diet has gotten sick and/or hated the process and gained more weight in the long run.

It is however the nature of the 5:2 Diet to count calories because it is vital that you do not accidentally cheat on fasting days. If you eat more than 25% of your normal daily caloric intake, your success on the 5:2 Diet will be severely cut back. That 25% limit on fasting days is the very maximum limit. If you can get by with eating less, on those days, you will lose weight and gain the health benefits from intermittent fasting more quickly. And yet, I am not encouraging you to eat less than 25% of your normal caloric intake but I am demanding – if I may! – that you never go over 25% those two days and the only way to ensure that is to count your calories.

So for the 5:2 Diet, I am modifying my typical don't-count-calories mantra. You *must* count them to ensure that your fasting days don't turn into cheat days accidentally.

Given the importance of exact calorie measurements, knowing that the calories in healthy oils and good proteins count less when it comes to increasing your waistline than starchy carbohydrate-based calories, on your non-fasting days feel free to eat more food than you might normally eat as long as it consists of healthy fats and good proteins. In other words, you are not actually binging on those days as long as the extra calories over what you might normally eat now primarily come from those two sources of food: healthy fats and proteins. In other words, I am giving you a back-door way to cheat on your non-fasting days. If you want to eat seven meals on the days that you don't fast, as long as those meals have healthy fats and healthy proteins, you are good to go.

But the one thing you need to do is *not* base your 25% of your daily calories on those extra fat and protein calories. In other words, simply take food that you normally eat now seven days a week, average out the number of calories that that would consist of, and use 25% of *that* for your two fasting day caloric limits. This means that you will be helping yourself because in effect you will be eating less than 25% of the calories you eat on the other days. But you will be eating 25% of the calories you eat currently. It's just that when you start the 5:2 Diet, you will eat more on non-fasting days and that "more" will be extremely healthy for you because it will consist of healthy fats and good proteins.

Note: Not to pat myself on the back, but I have yet to see any book on the 5:2 Diet discuss this issue of good fats and good proteins. They all seem to be primarily a caloric intake-based training manual. That not only does little to help your actual health, it can cause some people to binge on non-fasting days cannibalizing some of what happens on the fasting days.

12
THE SCIENCE BEHIND I.F.

So far you have learned about fasting, both through the 1-Day Diet as well as the 5:2 Diet. Before getting deeper into the specifics of the 5:2 Diet, let's take a short time-out to see what a doctor has to say about 5:2 Diet and related intermittent fasting (I.F.) routines.

We all seem to do better if we understand some of the process behind what is recommended. I don't want to waste your time with information you don't need. In reality, you do not have to understand how an engine works to drive a car well. At the same time, there's something funny about us when we go on a diet. We seem to focus so much on the diet that we begin to see reasons why it's not working at the time, and we begin to rationalize why it may be better to stop for a while and do something else.

Hence, our lack of success.

I want to give you just a little of the science behind intermittent fasting for the fundamental reason that I believe you will be more successful at sticking to the 5:2 Diet if you understand why, from a doctor's view point, intermittent fasting has the properties that it has. As I said earlier, nobody understands fully why intermittent fasting seems to have the benefits that it does. But it is a major research topic right now at many companies and in many labs for life extension, weight loss, and health benefits.

This means that we will see more and more about intermittent fasting, learn more about why it works, learn even better ways to approach it, and gain an understanding into ways to circumvent any of the problems that a few people rarely have with intermittent fasting; primarily excess hunger on fasting days.

You will be more successful with a "reason why." Below are some basics and I'll also present conclusions from an expert whom I greatly respect, Dr. Joseph Mercola.

Three Ways I.F. Benefits Health

By going a little longer without eating, you improve several health factors that can impact your body in major ways.

Insulin Sensitivity

Insulin is a hormone produced by your pancreas. The type of food you eat determines how much insulin your pancreas produces. Insulin determines the way our body uses or stores food.

Your insulin balance is critical to keep in check. Too little insulin, even in patients who do not have actual type 1 diabetes, can result in these problems:[37]

- Underweight

- Excess urination and bladder pressure due to increased thirst cravings

- Breathing problems dizziness

- Too much insulin, even in patients who do not have actual type 2 diabetes, can result in these problems, which often are the mirror images of type 1 diabetes:

- Obesity (obesity can also be part of the cause of type 2 diabetes)

- Menstrual abnormalities

- Depression and fatigue

- Low sex drives

If you are diagnosed with either type 1 or type 2 diabetes, you are probably going to require medical treatment to some degree or another for a long time and perhaps your entire life. Fortunately, many find that diet can help balance the insulin production and diabetes patients have found that proper diets can help reduce the negative effects and the severity of the disease... and get rid of it.

For our purposes, fasting, or even intermittent fasting, increases insulin sensitivity. This helps slow disease as well as the aging process, which is one reason fasting has been shown to increase longevity of life.

Oxidation[38]

Antioxidants help to fight cancer and keep your cells healthy. The berries I suggested that you put atop your list of healthy fruits are loaded with antioxidants. As with insulin sensitivity protection, fasting decreases the oxidation damage rate that is a natural process as we age. There is no way to live with our bodies forever; even the healthiest among us will some day pass away due to our bodies finally breaking down through oxidation and related cell-stress if not from disease or an accident.

Still, our quality of life as well as the longevity at which we live can directly be influenced by the rate of oxidation in our cells. Fasting can decrease this oxidation rate, which directly leads to a slowing of our aging process. In addition, the slower oxidization is said to help reduce our chances of getting cancer and is said to decrease the effects of cancer if we happen to get it.

Immunity

Our immune systems work full-time to protect us from outside attacks.[39] These attacks come from other people who are sick and carrying transmittable diseases. Immunity attacks can also come from our environment such as industrial chemicals, toxins in our food and water supplies, and by the perfectly normal process of aging, which reduces our immunity powers.

Note: If we had no immunity, the very first time we were exposed to a cold or flu or regular, naturally occurring toxin in the air, we would die. The more immune we are to our bodies' enemy infections, the less likely we are to pick up "bugs" here and there. This is why a strong immunity system is so critical to maintain.

If you exercise, your body improves. For example, if you perform weight-bearing exercises, you get stronger. This is because our bodies are extremely smart systems in that when they break down, they try to guard against that from happening in the future by building back up even stronger. Fasting has been shown to provide a similar result in that cells built during a fast will attempt to rebuild more strongly than the cells they replace which were stressed due to the fast.

This cell stressing is important for our health and is a good thing not a bad thing. Healthy foods such as organic broccoli provide nutrients and minerals that help our bodies and yet many people have no idea *why* they help. They help because foods that we see as healthy, such as fibrous, colorful, organic vegetables, will not only add nutrients to our diets but they also exercise our cells. That stress on certain cells in our bodies that fibrous, colorful vegetables cause will rebuild them in a stronger way.

Again, fasting mimics the same cellular behavior. Cells during a fast will be replaced by cells that are slightly stronger in order to hold up better under the next fast.

I.F. and Weight Loss

George Dvorsky has studied various intermittent fasting routines at length. He offers some interesting conclusions about the results, both from a health standpoint (some of which I touched on above) as well as intermittent fasting's pronounced ability to aid in weight loss[40]:

"... intermittent fasting (in this case, alternate-day fasting) lowers the chances of acquiring diabetes, while also lowering fasting glucose and insulin concentrations — and at rates comparable to caloric restriction.

"...Short-term fasting can induce growth hormone secretion in men (which is a problem for guys after they hit 30), it reduces oxidative stress (fasting prevents oxidative damage to cellular proteins by decreasing the accumulation of oxidative radicals in the cell — what contributes to aging and disease onset), and it's good for brain health, mental well-being, and clarity.

"And as a study published just last week has shown, restricting calories can also lengthen telomeres — which has a protective effect on our DNA and genetic material, which in turn helps with cellular health (i.e. it helps us extend healthy lifespan).

"And for people who wish to maintain a ketogenic diet — a metabolic state in which the body is in a perpetual state of fat burning instead of carbohydrate burning — intermittent fasting is a good way to help the body stay in ketosis."

The reason low-carbohydrate diets work is precisely because they enable the body to stay in a state of *ketosis* – which is a fat-burning mode – far longer than other diets. Not everybody can adapt to a low-carb diet, although it does seem to be an extremely healthy eating plan. Those people who cannot adapt to a low-carb lifestyle can achieve the same ketosis effect it appears through intermittent fasting.

Dr. Mercola Looks at I.F.

When I first heard about the 5:2 Diet, I began my in-depth research. Dr. Mercola quickly gets straight to the point as to why the 5:2 Diet, which is nothing more than intermittent fasting on a schedule and quantitative amount, works so well:

"Is it a good idea to 'starve' yourself just a little bit each day? The evidence suggests that yes, avoiding eating around the clock could have a very beneficial impact on your health and longevity.

"...It takes about six to eight hours for your body to metabolize your glycogen stores and after that you start to shift to burning fat. However, if you are replenishing your glycogen by eating every eight hours (or sooner), you make it far more difficult for your body to use your fat stores as fuel.

"It's long been known that restricting calories in certain animals can increase their lifespan by as much as 50 percent, but more recent research suggests that sudden and intermittent calorie restriction appears to provide the same health benefits as constant calorie restriction, which may be helpful for those who cannot successfully reduce their everyday calorie intake (or aren't willing to).

"Unfortunately, hunger is a basic human drive that can't be easily suppressed, so anyone attempting to implement serious calorie restriction is virtually guaranteed to fail. Fortunately you don't have to deprive yourself as virtually all of the benefits from calorie restriction can be achieved through properly applied intermittent fasting."[1]

Dr. Mercola discusses non-weight issues that see benefits from intermittent fasting when he describes the following problems addressed to some degree or another by intermittent fasting:

- High cholesterol
- High blood sugar (related to the insulin issues I mentioned earlier)

- Fatty liver disease[42]
- Metabolic problems (your body's ability to burn fat and create muscle)[43]

Constantly eating three (or more) full meals a day with snacks in between never gives your body enough time to regenerate cells well.[44] When your body digests food, your stomach consumes a large amount of resources. This is why when you eat a lot of food you tend to get tired. Your body literally is trying to put you to sleep to free up some energy to digest all that food.

All your life you have probably heard the phrase, "breakfast is the most important meal of the day." Actually, the repeatable results of intermittent fasting sure seem counteract that statement.

Some forms of intermittent fasting, such as eating only between 12 noon and 8 PM, show dramatic improvements in several health factors such as those I've mentioned so far. It seems as though our bodies are still trying to digest our evening meal, absorb any nutrients from our food, and eliminate toxins, activities which occur in a big way during sleep and during the hours after we wake up. When we get up and eat immediately in the mornings, we put a halt to all of that activity still going on and start it all over again before the last phase of last night's process has ended.

Eating without ever fasting, and keep in mind that intermittent fasting shows near-identical results to long-term fasts, so eating *without* ever fasting keeps our bodies' motors always going, always working, and in many ways never completing the tasks that our bodies begin. This has got to put stress on our bodies. This has got to decrease our lifespan because, as with a motor that is used too much without being allowed to cool, our bodies simply get worn out faster than they would if they had a chance to regenerate once in a while.

Intermittent fasting seems to be one of the easiest ways to allow our bodies to do that regeneration.

The regeneration happens at a cell level and over time our cells all replaced each other. As we age, eat the wrong foods consistently, never fast, and never exercise, that cell replacement does still take place, but there is nothing to make our cells regenerate stronger than the cells they are replacing. Our cells either get replaced with identical cells or, as we age, inferior cells.

Dr. Mercola concludes with this:

"This suggests that your body may benefit from the break it receives while fasting, whereas constant eating may lead to metabolic exhaustion and health consequences like weight gain. Researchers said their latest work shows it's possible to stave off metabolic disease by simply restricting when you eat with periodic fasting, or even by just keeping to regular meal schedules rather than 'grazing' off and on all day. They concluded:

"[Time-restricted feeding] is a nonpharmacological strategy against obesity and associated diseases."

When You Should *Not* Perform I.F.

Dr. Mercola does have one warning against intermittent fasting:

"As for pregnant and/or lactating women, I don't think fasting would be a wise choice. Your baby needs plenty of nutrients, during and after birth, and there's no research supporting fasting during this important time. On the contrary, some studies suggest it might be contraindicated, as it can alter fetal breathing patterns, heartbeat, and increase gestational diabetes. It may even induce premature labor. I don't think it's worth the risk.

"Instead, my recommendation would be to really focus on improving your nutrition during this crucial time. A diet with plenty of raw organic, biodynamic foods, and foods high in healthful fats, coupled with high quality proteins will give your baby a head start on good health. You'll also want to be sure to include plenty of cultured and fermented foods to optimize your — and consequently your baby's — gut flora."

What About the Heart?

According to the Centers for Disease Control and Prevention, coronary problems – heart disease – is the number one cause of death in the USA. Keep in mind heart-based technology has improved dramatically over the last 100 years. Once people are diagnosed with heart problems, technology can do a lot to diagnose their symptoms and save their lives.

The problem is the presence of heart disease to begin with. Heart disease is a *new problem*. Isn't that a surprise?

Did you know that in 1920 when Paul Dudley White invented the electrocardiograph[45] (the precursor to the electrocardiogram, the EKG or ECG), his Harvard colleagues suggested that he abandon that invention and work on a more "profitable branch of medicine"?[46]

Heart disease and related problems such as hypertension were statistically not even on the radar. Heart disease occurred in such few people it wasn't worth focusing on as recently as the 1920s. We must admit we are a failure at so many aspects in nutrition, medicine, and prevention.

But intermittent fasting offers a possible heartfelt solution!

The Big News Network recently reported the following:

"Fasting twice a week could be the key to a longer life by slashing the risk of a host of killer diseases, a new study has revealed. Research shows dramatically cutting the amount of calories you eat for two days can keep obesity, heart disease and diabetes at bay, the Daily Express reported.

"Researchers have backed... intermittent fasting and say it is as effective as weight loss surgery, without the cost or risk. ...

"Scientists say it [intermittent fasting] has some cardiovascular benefits that appear similar to exercising, such as improving blood pressure and heart rate and lowering cholesterol."

The study described above, a review of intermittent fasting diets published by the British

Journal of Diabetes and Vascular Disease, by a team led by James Brown from Aston University, states: intermittent fasting not only affects the waistline, metabolism, insulin sensitivity, and so forth, but unexpectedly to most of us, it also improves our *cardiovascular functioning*, and does so basically *as well as exercise* if we are to believe their conclusions.

This leads me to think that intermittent fasting is the future of dieting. It's not a fad.

13
5:2 FAT-BURNING – INEXPENSIVE *AND* CUSTOMIZABLE

Let's face it. Most people go on a diet such as the 5:2 Diet, not for health reasons but to lose weight. We would all love to be healthier, but we all *really* want to look good...!

A website devoted to intermittent fasting, called *The IF Life* all about intermittent fasting, eating, and fitness[47] has some interesting information on the fat-burning properties of intermittent fasting. But what I like about the site is that it never forgets that intermittent fasting-based eating plans, such as the 5:2 Diet, saves you money as well as being healthy and helps you to lose weight. You will spend less money each week for food than you otherwise would if you were eating three (or more) full meals each day along with snacks and so forth.

The Downsides Are Few and Far Between

There is very little downside to a diet based on intermittent fasting. And unless your doctor tells you not to, or unless you're pregnant, the 5:2 Diet and the alternatives that we will discuss shortly appear to be amazingly effective not only in helping people get healthier and lose weight, but also save money, and put less emphasis on food.

This enables you, when you *do* eat, especially on non-fasting days on special occasions you will find that when you do eat, even though you are not famished, you will appreciate your food more and enjoy it more! It's almost as though the resetting of your digestion system on fasting days, enables you to go back to a Ground Zero when it comes to food and taste. You seem to enjoy the flavors of food more and you will appreciate food more all at the same time as not feeling deprived on fasting days.

Customizing the 5:2 for You

The 5:2 Diet is extremely simple, so much so that within the first few pages you knew virtually all of the requirements for it. The only thing left is to learn some details, which will help answer questions and will confirm that the 5:2 Diet may be right for you.

At this point, you have those details. You know, for example:

- What to do two days a week (fast, eating 25% of your normal caloric levels)

- What to do five days a week (eating whatever you want, without pigging out, while understanding that if you limit starchy carbs such as corn, potatoes, and whole grains, as well as sweets including most fruit, that your results will be much quicker if you use good judgment most of the time on those five days)

- Why the 5:2 Diet - which is just one form of intermittent fasting - helps you lose weight

- Why the 5:2 Diet helps protect your body from diseases

- Why the 5:2 Diet offers longevity improvements related to how long you possibly can live

The Modifications

Feel free to modify the 5:2 Diet. If you have absolutely no problem eating only 25% of your normal levels two days a week, you might try going a week or two on a 4:3 Diet modification. The benefits of that greater intermittent fasting routine, which as you know by now means a reduction in the amount of digestion your body has to perform, should improve all of the health benefits and amplify the weight loss results from being on the 5:2 Diet where you follow intermittent fasting routines only two days a week.

If you cannot follow this requirement to eat 25% of your food three days a week; that is okay. This is simply one form of modifying the concept of the 5:2 Diet.

Note: The 5:2 Diet is more of a concept than an actual diet. Yes, as you know the five and the two are critical elements of the actual 5:2 Diet as it is known throughout the health and dieting world. But there is nothing magical about eating two days a week 25% less than you eat the other five. The "magic" if you will, is in the intermittent fasting and not in the number of times or days you do that.

Trial and Error – Vacations and Such

Trial and error may be the best way to find what is best for you. Trial and error may be the best way to find which specific details of the 5:2 Diet *concept* works for you and your lifestyle. For example, if you're going on vacation for five days, you may very well not want to fast on any of those five days. That's fine.

The 1-Day Diet is truly the simplest way to prepare yourself a day ahead of trouble and to fix yourself the day after you get back from a vacation. So do the 1-Day Diet the day before the vacation and the day after you get back from vacation.

Other Alternatives to Consider

Often people writing about the 5:2 Diet discuss the alternative of a *6:1 Diet.* By now you should have little problem guessing what such an alternative might consist of: You eat 25% of your normal caloric intake one day a week and eat normally the other six.

On a 6:1 Diet schedule, you obviously will lose weight more slowly than the 5:2 Diet and 4:3 Diet version. Still, some people simply cannot handle a 5:2 Diet intermittent fasting schedule, even though it means they only have to spend two days each week eating three small meals.

There is absolutely nothing wrong with moving to a 6:1 Diet schedule if it works for you, and if the 5:2 Diet does not work for you for any reason whatsoever.

In three months you may lose only as much weight on a 6:1 Diet schedule as you might lose in a single month on the 5:2 Diet schedule. But who cares? That is still success in anybody's book! Let me say, I have tried the 6:1 Diet, and it was so simple for me that I did not want to stay on it. I wanted to move immediately to the 5:2 Diet to see the effects that it had on me. But if I were unable to maintain two days a week with 25% of my normal calories, I would have immediately gone back to the 6:1 Diet and still written this book based on my results personally and on my research.

Again, I think my own long-term experience with my 10-Hour Coffee Diet and 1-Day Diet plans make it far easier for me to adopt the 5:2 Diet plan for several months so that I can discuss the plan properly with you here. But this will not be true for everybody, and yet I do think that it would be rare that someone could not easily follow a 6:1 Diet routine.

Why a Diet?

The reason I avoid the term diet in most of my books on health and nutrition is because people often view a diet as a short-term eating regimen instead of a lifelong eating plan. The benefits of intermittent fasting, which you will gain from the 5:2 Diet plan and alternatives, are not benefits that you get once and then you can stop worrying about them. A lifelong intermittent fasting plan is a perfectly good eating routine for life.

Food-restriction studies have shown conclusively, that a food restrictive diet, whether that restriction comes in the form of time, amount of food, or both as in the 5:2 Diet, can be followed for life to extend the effects of such an eating plan and to amplify all of its benefits. Unless you have stomach problems, are pregnant, or your doctor informs you that an eating routine that consists of intermittent fasting may be dangerous specifically for you for whatever reason, there appears to be absolutely no destructive effects from such a diet.

Don't think of the 1-Day Diet or the 5:2 Diet as a "diet" even though "diet is included in the name.

Think instead of the 5:2 Diet (or whatever alternative you find that works best for you) as being a lifelong eating plan for you. Sure there will be times, such as vacation or sickness, when you overeat on days you should be fasting, or under eat on days that you should be eating normally, but generally if you can keep your intermittent fasting plan working for life, you should feel far better consistently than you otherwise would and no health consequences of its long-term, lifelong use should arise.

14
MAKING THE 5:2 DIET EVEN EASIER!

Once you find the eating plan that fits you best, related to the 5:2 Diet concept of intermittent fasting, all sorts of ways exist to make the 5:2 Diet concept even easier.

For an example, on your fasting days as well as your non-fasting days, you can have all the tea and coffee you like. If you use sweetener in these drinks, stick with Stevia. Stevia is an all-natural sweetener that comes directly from a plant. Don't use sugar, not even cane or "raw" sugar, on your fasting days and try to avoid it on your non-fasting days two.

> **Note:** Tea and coffee are grown in regions where numerous pesticides are used. Make sure you always buy organic coffee and tea. In addition, a study recently showed that tea bags can contain a surprising amount of toxins and cancerous compounds. If you steep tea, buy organic loose tea and use a stainless steel tea strainer instead of using tea bags.[48]

I have been using Stevia now for several years and love it. Stevia has no impact on your glycemic index, which means it has zero effect on your hips, thighs, and belly! In addition, Stevia actually can fight plaque on your gum lines. I was shocked to hear how many people use Stevia on their toothbrushes instead of toothpaste that often contains dangerous fluoride.

What About Vitamins?

There's an amazingly powerful option, but know up front that it can be a little expensive. You can use a powerful vitamin and mineral liquid to replace one of your fasting meals. I've found that *IntraMax* is so powerful most people absolutely do not feel hungry for at least 3 and a half hours. The 71 organic trace minerals, the 17 essential fatty acids, the 33 super green foods, the 14 seeds and sprouts, and the 80 vitamin sources in every ounce insures that you won't go hungry and that your health is not compromised when you eat less.

I realize this sounds like an ad, but I need you to know that I did not get anything for telling you about this product other than my own satisfaction that I have let others know about what is perhaps the very best single supplement ever made. IntraMax is high-priced because it is perhaps the best made in the world as far as a multi-nutritional complex organic food supplement. And given that it is a meal replacement for me, it actually costs very little since you're not spending money on food that you would otherwise eat.

You can get IntraMax from DruckerLabs: (http://store.druckerlabs.com/intraMAXinfo _s/117.htm)

Note: Good things are not always simple or cheap. You cannot order IntraMax directly unless you have a medical practice of some kind or are certified in health and nutrition. Your doctor however can order the product without a problem. Remember that each one-ounce serving contains only 64 calories.

Expand the 5:2 Diet with Spices and a Delicious Green Smoothie (And a Secret Eating Tip)

I want to repeat something I said earlier in passing and then take a page or two to expound upon it in light of the 5:2 Diet:

"... good food, real food, food that is good for your body, is not boring or bland food! Those who understand how to eat well also understand the importance of spices. Spices are the underutilized secret of good food and nutrition. There's a reason why history books are filled with centuries of explorers and pirates hunting for the best spice routes in the medieval world. It's because only recently with the prevalence of processed, pre-packed non-'food' have we forgotten what makes food taste good. Spices make food taste good."

You need to use more spices. On the 5:2 Diet, spices become an extraordinary treat that add incredible tastes to your food *without adding one significant calorie to your fasting days!*

In the USA, and in most countries in the West, spices are underutilized dramatically. We are finding that our brains are not developing as well without spices as they do with spices! Spices work to improve our bodies regulating functions. For example, cinnamon helps reduce the impact of starchy carbohydrates. So if you eat ice cream, sprinkling cinnamon on top of the ice cream helps reduce the fattening effects of that ice cream.

Spices and Health

Not only are many spices great for your brain's health and your body's balance but they do two things:

- They give food more taste
- They stack the advantages of an already healthy diet![49]

In other words, once you begin to eat well, if you then add spices to your food the advantages of those good foods will be multiplied by the spices. You will lose weight *faster* if you eat a healthy, low-carb diet *with* spices such as cayenne pepper and turmeric than if you do not include those spices.

> **Note:** Eating a half-teaspoon of red chili flakes before a meal, for example, is said to decrease the average caloric intake by about 15%. That 15% adds up over time to a lot of calories that your body and brain don't have to deal with.

Spices and herbs maximize nutrient density. They create a more thermogenic diet[50] and make you younger and healthier due to their medicinal-like properties. Spices can increase your feeling of fullness so you'll eat less, and helps you to eliminate adding too much phony, unhealthy "spices" such as bleached table salt, High Fructose Corn Syrup-based ketchup, worthless pre-ground cardboard called "pepper," and other awful condiments to your meals.

This feeling of being full, by using spices to your advantage, is especially important to someone on the 5:2 Diet. On fasting days, the spices will give you a more complete feeling without adding any calories to your meals. You will be improving the burning effects of your body's metabolism, your food will taste far better, you will enjoy your meals more, and you will feel full with less food.

I am surprised most diet books don't discuss the benefits of adding in spices.

The 5:2 Green Smoothie

I don't want to turn this into a cookbook with 100's of recipes you can use for the 5:2 Diet. That's not the purpose here. There are many cookbooks on the market that take care of that if you want specific 5:2 Diet recipes.

But I did want to add this one recipe. The difference between a green smoothie and a traditional smoothie is that a green smoothie uses vegetables with a *little* fruit for taste often tossed in. More traditional smoothies are fruit-based (think *Jamba Juice*) or more dessert-based such as chocolate peanut-butter smoothies are little more than a chocolate peanut-butter milkshake with the name changed to make it sound healthier.

When you throw vegetables into the drink, especially when the smoothie is primarily comprised of vegetables, it's far healthier than the other two without all the sugar and fructose.

> **Note:** If you're a smoothie lover then you know how bananas can help a smoothie not only taste good but it adds a nice texture that you might miss if you omit bananas from your diet. (And I suggest you do omit them; bananas are a high-glycemic natural food that can pack on the pounds by turning to sugar very fast.) Instead of a banana put half an avocado in your smoothie! It adds a similar texture and actually improves the taste quite a bit if you've got berries and green veggies in the mix already, as you almost certainly will have with healthy green smoothies.

Recipes for green smoothies are easy because all you need are the ingredients! Just put them in a blender and you're good to go.

To make a delicious 5:2 Green Smoothie, put these in your blender and mix it up:

- 1 cup kale or spinach
- Pinch of parsley
- 1/2 small avocado
- 1/2 tbsp cinnamon
- 1/4 cup mixed berries
- 1 cup chilled coconut water or water
- 1/2 cup ice
- 1 tbsp lemon juice
- Pinch of cayenne (unless you do not like this spice)

Total calories: About 180, perfect for one of your three fasting meals!

Secret Eating Tip

Want to know how to extend the amount of time that you eat nothing while at the same time increase the amount of food you can eat for your 5:2 Diet fast meals?

It is simple, and maybe you thought of it earlier, but here it is: if possible, wait until noon for your first meal on fasting days. If you are like most people, you won't find this difficult. This not only improves your systems digestion and detoxification by extending the cleanup work your body did during the night by several hours after you awake, but it also means that when you finally can eat at noon you can have a larger meal. Instead of eating only 25% of the number of calories you normally would eat at three meals, your noon meal can be a third more due to only eating 2 meals instead of 3 meals on your fasting day.

An Eating Example

Let's go back to numbers I used earlier and consider them in light of the sample recipes in the previous chapter.

Assume you're female and normally try to eat 2,200 calories each day on regular, non-fasting days. This means that on fasting days you can eat a total of only 550 calories. This limits the calories you can have at each meal to a paltry 184 calories.

But if you eat your first meal at noon, and have only one additional meal that day, each meal can be up to 275 calories.

The 5:2 Diet Cheat Sheet is a *Pattern* of Answers

Yes, it is true that you will either need to devise your own 5:2 Diet meals or find a 5:2 Diet cookbook. But the purpose of this 5:2 Diet Cheat Sheet was not to give you an exhaustive list of possible food to eat, but its goal is, rather to give you *patterns* of what to do.

You can go to your frozen food aisle at any grocery store, and buy a generic, low calorie, frozen meal that will have the vitamins and nutrients of the cardboard it comes in. It also will taste like the cardboard comes in, and you will grow tired of such food quickly. While it's true that you only fast twice a week, and since your fast days are nonconsecutive days you will rarely get tired of them. At the same time, I want you to go into this with a huge chance at success. Not just success, I want you to enjoy the 5:2 Diet. In order to enjoy it, and therefore stick with it, and possibly stick with it for the rest of your life, you need to eat food that is delicious, as well as healthy.

Nutrient dense food will fill you up on less calories, keep you healthier, and offer a far higher success rate when you begin the 5:2 Diet. So my pattern for the 5:2 Diet has been trying to teach you ways to approach this that not only will work for you since you can customize everything, but also that works best for your body.

Oh, and here's another quick tip you can use on the two fasting days. Consider eating protein bars. But with those, be careful with the calories. Be sure to read the labels on the protein bars so you don't get too many calories (or sugar). Most protein bars are notorious for being glorified candy bars. But there are still some good ones out there.

Section 3:

STUPID Hormones!
The Hormone Weight Loss Solution

—

Fix Your CRAZY Hormones
and Finally
Lose Weight for Good!

15
INTRODUCTION TO HORMONES AND HEALTH

We've all ridden the diet merry-go-round. Some of us have done so far too many times.

Round and round we go, and when we stop we're back to the weight we began... or higher.

If you're tried diet after diet you're not alone. Powerful diets such as the 1-Day Diet and the 5:2 Diets will not be as effective if your hormones are out of whack.

But it is possible to be healthy, be fit, and feel great. That is, *if* you understand that your hormones are the regulators that work for you or against you. Hormones stop your weight loss or add to your weight loss. They keep you healthy or allow you to deteriorate. As your hormones go so goes your health.

If you want to understand a better approach than a diet merry-go-round, you've come to the right place.

Jennifer Jolan & Rich Bryda

16
HEALTH IS THE KEY, NOT WEIGHT

The key to losing weight and *keeping* it off is not found in any diet on earth. The key to losing weight and *keeping* it off isn't any eating plan in existence today.

The key to losing weight and keeping it off is two-fold:

1. Fix your health

2. Live a healthy lifestyle

Your body is a regulating machine. Your body knows its optimum weight. In spite of bad weight experiences you've maybe had in the past, your body *does* always want to get to its optimum weight as quickly as it can. A well-oiled machine works tirelessly and when your body is the equivalent of a well-oiled machine it will work for you in ways you never dreamed. But until you oil it – that is, until you fix your health and adopt a lifelong healthy eating and health regimen – your body is not going to be able to work with you. Your body will work against you.

The result of our bodies working against us is the overweight condition we often find ourselves in. This multiplies into severe health problems later. We focus too much on the symptom and not the real problem. The problem is not the fat stored on our thighs, hips, and around our waists. Our bodies simply don't have the ability to stay at an optimum weight when we don't correct our control center.

Do you know what your body uses to control weight loss or weight gain? Your body uses the same mechanisms to control your weight that it uses to control how you feel at any given moment, how you look, how your skin feels, how active you are, how much sex you desire, how much you sleep, how effectively you think and communicate, and scores of other factors. Primarily, your body uses hormones as triggers to turn on and off every aspect of your well-being.

We're going to help you balance your hormones and health. Maximizing your hormones *before* focusing on weight loss will produce results you might find amazing. Once you fix your hormones, weight loss will be an easy and a natural result. Treat the problem (your messed up hormones) and not the symptoms (your extra weight).

> **Note:** Sometimes, malnutrition and bad brain nutrients and imbalanced hormones can put you into a state of starvation even though you are eating a lot. If you are underweight and want to bump up your pounds, don't focus on eating more. Focus on getting your brain and hormones, your body's central control panel switches, where they should be. Your body will then be freed up to get your weight to a more optimal level.

By the way, as you begin to stabilize your hormones to healthy levels, your weight will not be the first thing to be fixed by your newly healthy body. Your digestion, sleep patterns, energy levels, and strength will probably improve first. After your body has adjusted properly to its new turbo-charged hormone levels the weight will begin to drop consistently.

Hormones Control Your Health, Your Brain Controls Your Hormones and Other Things

To put yourself into the best shape you've ever been, you *must* focus on your body's regulators. Those are your key hormones that need to be in balance.

There is another factor to consider too. Besides your hormones, you must also get your brain into balance, as mentioned in our 10-Hour Coffee Diet book. Even if you consider yourself a clear thinker, that doesn't mean that your brain's nutrients are in their optimal state and balance. Your brain actively controls your various body's reactions and hormone triggers.

When you have an imbalance in your brain's primary chemicals and neurotransmitters, you must correct that imbalance immediately. Otherwise your brain won't be fully freed up to handle what it was designed to do. If you're overweight and tired, an out-of-balance brain needs to be looked into and fixed first before focusing on pure weight loss. If you don't, your weight loss will be temporary at best and can possibly work *against* your overall health.

It's critical that you focus both on your brain's chemical nutrients and your body's hormone balances, together. For decades, books, trainers, and nutritionists have focused on the symptom – being overweight – and not the regulators and controllers of the symptom – hormones and the brain's chemical nutrients. Recent revelations about the brain and hormone balances have produced astounding results when it comes to people's health and weight levels.

It's so very true that we cannot emphasize it enough: Fix your hormones and brain nutrients and you'll fix your health… *and* lose weight! Lucky for you, the 1-Day Diet helps fix your hormones.

When Things Are Severe

Obviously, some people have severe health problems that must be addressed immediately, such as Multiple Sclerosis and Alzheimer's issues. We are not saying that bringing the hormones and brain back into balance will fix those overnight or ever.

But so many times, the symptoms of those severe diseases and other maladies such as hypertension and high cholesterol can be caused by hormone imbalances. At the very least, hormone, brain nutrient, vitamin, and mineral deficiencies can contribute to the start of such maladies and are even instrumental in keeping those problems active.

No matter where you are on the healthy/unhealthy meter, if you repair your hormones you will at the *least* begin to stop contributing to other problems hampered by hormone imbalances. And at best you may see reversals. Your hormones will be able once again to regulate your body and your brain will once again be able to regulate your hormones and other activities.

Hormonal Balance is Pure Health

If you fail to believe that serious issues *can* be addressed through a non-medicinal look at your body, your hormones, your brain, and your lifestyle, you owe it to yourself to watch the following astounding video by Dr. Terry Wahls.[51] A few years ago, her Multiple Sclerosis reached the tipping point so much so that her MS confined her to a wheelchair for four years until she began systematically reversing her MS and actually repaired her brain's myelin sheathing (the insulation around the brain's pathways).

Her video is here (and if you know anything about MS this will amaze you): http://kaleu niversity.org/5103-multiple-sclerosis-dr-wahls

Dr. Wahls now spends her days bike-riding and skiing and has been symptom-free from MS just 18 months after focusing on a non-medicinal lifestyle which fixed her brain, hormones, and MS through diet alone. Remember, she was an invalid just a couple of years earlier, confined to a wheelchair without a decent quality of life.

The FDA, USDA, AMA, AOA, and all the others in the governmental and medical community seem to have a big interest in keeping drug promotions going and not promote nutrition and preventive maintenance that helps keep problems away before they begin. That is why we leave it up to Dr. Wahls to convince you in her video.

Always remember: if you focus on food and weight without the vision of fixing your body's control systems, you may lose weight temporarily but your body is going to halt your weight loss eventually and revert back to storing weight. Your body simply won't have the ability or freedom to regulate your weight properly.

Stop Your Moans By Fixing Your Hormones

It turns out that if you want real results to appear on your hips and thighs you must take care of your body's regulators. Those are your hormones! Ultimately, the health of your body depends on the health of your hormones.

Sure, it's possible to starve yourself by reducing your ingested calories down to an extremely low level and you'll lose weight. Maybe. For a while at least. You lose weight because you literally starve your body and it must begin to cannibalize itself including your muscles and whatever lean tissue mass you happen to have. But on most calorie-restrictive lifestyles you and your health will go away as quickly as the fat. Only the fat will return.

You must make a promise to yourself: Assuming we convince you that the proper hormones fuel produces the best body results possible, and we will, your goal from this point forward should be to focus not on your thighs but on your hormones *first*.

To lose weight and build lean muscle mass, get more energy, and feel better, it's not always about fixing your caloric intake.

To the extent you've happened to balance some hormones in the past through eating, you may have accomplished some of those goals. Nevertheless, since you didn't realize the prime importance of focusing on your hormone regulators first then you didn't accomplish your goals as fully as you could have. And if you're like most of us, you didn't stay lean or feel good for long. Because you weren't taught that your hormones are the regulators of how much you weigh and how good you feel.

Weight control isn't about calories – weight control is all about hormones.

17
WHAT EXACTLY IS A HORMONE?

If you've read anything about hormones in the past you may have been left with more questions than answers. One of the reasons so many people get confused when told about hormones is that the fundamentals aren't explained. Until you understand the basics, you have less reason to accept or believe that hormone balance will play such a large role in your health and weight loss.

It's the goal of this section of the 1-Day Diet book to make hormones as easy to understand as possible. You don't need to know microbiology to understand the fundamentals of hormones. You don't need a degree in Health Sciences to realize how vital hormones are to every aspect of your body. We aren't going to go in-depth into charts and graphs and diagrams of the functions of hormones.

Who cares about all that if you're not in school? You just want to know how to get healthy and achieve your optimum weight, right? All that takes is understand just the basics of hormones and then you need to learn ways to put your key hormones into balance.

Hormones 101

Let's keep this short, shall we? You want answers not science. Although the underlying science is actually fun for us, we don't want to waste your time. We want to give you answers that will balance key hormones and put your weight optimization into full gear.

The system in your body that contains your hormones is collectively called your *endocrine system.*[52]

A hormone is a chemical in your body. Usually, a hormone is created or generated in one part of your body by an organ and sent to another part of your body to do a job. Many hormones perform multiple jobs. Many of your body's hormones, or chemicals, can regulate multiple activities. Our glandular system is primarily responsible for hormone creation although we can generate some of our needed hormones elsewhere such as in our stomach. Our cells can produce hormones too, which then regulate other cells.

Examples of organs that can create hormones in bodies are:

- Ovaries

- Testes

- Thyroid Gland

- Pituitary Gland

The bottom line is this: a hormone is a specific chemical that helps regulate a part or parts of your body. The regulation might be physical such as sexual functioning or it might seem to be more of a chemical regulation such as metabolism.

Hormones allow for free-flowing or blocked communication and bodily responses. If you are low on a hormone, the organ or cells or chemical that hormone is supposed to regulate or communicate with will be out of balance and not work optimally.

Your body contains, produces, and acts upon many different hormones. Several hundred hormones run around in your system as a matter of fact. There is not one key hormone although some hormones play more important and active roles than others. In this book we will focus on the hormones that help the typical body get and stay healthy and get and stay lean.

Sources of Hormones

As said, your body usually creates hormones. A healthy, vibrant body creates a good balance of needed hormones.

Through various actions and sources such as supplementation and prescriptions you can add certain hormones to your body through non-natural means. This is not in and of itself bad although many sources and methods for increasing certain hormones have been flawed through the years. Some synthetic hormones are used in *hormone replacement therapy* effectively while others have been found to be dangerous and produce unexpected results.

A healthy body with all the right ingredients in place will generally produce a healthy array of hormones that work in tandem and are in balance. As we age, our hormone generation can decrease. This can be okay depending on the hormone and your response and needs. For others, adding back hormones as aging occurs can be a big benefit through synthetic hormone replacement or a newer method called bio-identical hormone replacement, which replace specific hormones with identical chemical structure to the same hormones created by your body as opposed to a synthetic hormone, which differs at the chemical level from a 100% naturally produced hormone.

Diseases find it far more difficult to manifest themselves in your body when your hormones are in balance. It can't be said enough times: focusing on hormonal balance, perhaps for the first time in your life, means you will be healthier and your weight will be far easier to control than if you let your hormones get out of balance.

A Quick Introductory Example

Not every hormone we're going to discuss here relates to weight loss directly, but they all relate indirectly in some way. For example, there is a hormone that regulates how well you sleep. If you aren't sleeping well, you'll learn ways to help improve that hormone's imbalance. The hormone is melatonin.

Melatonin is important because sleep is important for health reasons. A lack of sleep makes us less effective at work so our work suffers and ultimately our productivity can suffer from long-term insomnia enough to affect future advancement. Long-term fatigue makes us susceptible to illness through a deterioration of our immune systems.

The hormone melatonin is critical for weight loss even though melatonin's primary job is to regulate sleep. As the October 5, 2010 *Annals of Internal Medicine* explains, dieters who got adequate sleep lose twice the amount of body fat that they lost when their sleep was restricted. In addition, with inadequate amounts of sleep the dieters felt far hungrier due to an imbalance in the ghrelin hormone, a hormone that regulates hunger.

Given this initial example, when we cover hormones throughout this book that don't directly seem to impact your weight loss, please know that they do impact your weight loss *indirectly* at the very least. And don't you want to stack the odds in your favor every step of the way with losing weight? Don't you want to maximize and optimize your body's weight loss? Certainly you do and so all of the hormones discussed here play an important role in your health and weight. In addition, if a hormone relates to your body's overall health, such as your thyroid, there is no way your body is going to be able to focus on optimizing your weight if it's dealing with an imbalance in its thyroid.

Your body is an amazing, multi-processing machine that works on many activities at once. But your body can get stressed out when forced to deal with problem areas that you could otherwise eliminate. Balancing hormones is a required way to ensure that any excess weight is dealt with effectively and as quickly as possible.

Dysfunctional Hormones

Hormones act dysfunctional when they are out of balance or not at their peak levels. Not only do organs and cells not communicate with each other effectively when your hormones are not at their peak levels, but some low hormone levels cause poor nutrient uptake in your body so you don't get the nutrition your body needs to function properly.

Hormone overloads can cause as much damage or more than low levels of hormones.

For example, both estrogen and testosterone are present in healthy men and women. Obviously, the levels considered normal for one gender differs for the other gender.

Today we are experiencing far greater levels of estrogen due to pesticides in the soil and soy in food products. (Soy sauce is not a risk factor because the soy is fermented and doesn't cause the negative effects in men.) By the time you add up the amount of pesticides ingested from the non-organic foods we buy, we eat one pound of pesticides each year. From the start, the average American is being attacked with hormone-damaging food. We're going to be discussing food quite a bit in this book as well as food sources and the types of food that help align your hormonal balance instead of put your hormones out of sync.

The Bottom Line

Hormones control your sex drive. Hormones control how well you sleep. Hormones control your metabolism by determining whether food you eat should be used for energy right then or stored as fat. Hormones control when you are hungry and when you are full. If hormones regulate virtually every activity in your body including the ability or inability to lose weight, doesn't it make sense to get your hormones working at the best in order to get to your best weight possible?

Many diets address just one or two hormones whether or not they realize it. You need to concentrate on a series of primary hormones to help your health and then to lose weight and keep it off. Earlier in the 1-Day Diet, nothing was said about hormones. Yet, the diet is actually geared toward optimizing several key hormones and, using a few tricks, produces extremely quick results especially for those who have tried to lose weight in the past using more traditional calorie restrictive weight loss diets.

18
FOOD AND HORMONES

Sadly, many of our hormone problems come from man-made activities. It's not just a poor diet that can put our hormones out of balance. It's how we typically live as well.

The fault is not ours necessarily. Our society has become prosperous. Technology has developed new ways to do more with fewer resources. This prosperity comes with a price however. In getting more for less, in producing more using fewer resources, things slip along the way. Sadly, our health is often one of the casualties. The choices for lower-quality foods should still be available because some food is better than no food if you're starving. But the problem comes in when the food and drug companies all have financial incentives to keep you ignorant of good and bad choices.

The Food Supply

I talk a lot about organic food and I realize it can be costly. If you can't go organic for your produce, just start buying a few organic foods. Every little but helps. The term "organic" was unknown to our great-grandparents. They often grew most of what they ate. Their cattle and chickens and pigs were fed in part scraps from the table. The table scraps that they couldn't feed to the pigs they would put in a box outside to produce compost to enrich the soil in the next set of crops. They used their chicken coop's waste product to fertilize and enrich soil used for new plantings. They would rotate crops to maintain a healthy blend of nutrients in the soil. Often their produce was so high in nutrients that pesticides were hardly needed.

Note: When plants have a high nutritional value, often called a *high-brix reading*, bugs that would otherwise eat the plants get diarrhea and die because their systems don't handle highly nutritious produce well.

A fully functioning farm, sometimes today called a *permaculture* farm, utilized all resources in a closed system. Run-off water from one field was used to water another that was planted below it. The upper tier would need fresher water and the lower-tier getting the runoff had crops that grew better with the secondary water.

Organic and permaculture farming are buzzwords today that are treated as though they are some newfangled way of growing food. Your great grandparents didn't use the terms permaculture or organic or high-brix. They called it "farming" and "ranching" and "gardening."

Your great grandparents didn't worry about their food not being nutritious enough. It was nutritious enough.

Today, with the conventional foods we eat, we've paid the price in health problems that have become epidemic. Our hormones cannot keep up with the demands placed on them. Our bodies therefore cannot keep up.

Dr. Al Sears, MD, wrote this:[53]

[...] but today an apple a day is not going to do anything for you. The produce you get from your grocery store doesn't have the same level of vitamins, minerals or fiber it did years ago. In fact, you would have to eat 26 of today's apples to equal just one apple from 1914. (Source: Lindlahr, 1914: USDA 1963 and 1997.)

Why should you care about that? Commercial farming has stripped our food of the very nutrients we need to stay vital, young and full of energy.

Today's commercial farmers grow fruits and vegetables that are designed to look good on the shelf. That means they're often little more than pith and water. And harsh fertilizers leave the soil with few – if any – minerals to nourish the plants.

Even the U.S. Department of Agriculture admits that vitamin and mineral levels have fallen by as much as 81 percent over the last 30 years.

Genetics and Hormones in Our Foods

Perhaps you've heard of *GMO* food. This is *genetically modified organism* (sometimes called *genetically engineered organism* or *GEO*[54]). This is food that includes crops as well as animals that have been genetically modified.

The goal of all this phony food modification is to grow a larger food supply in a smaller amount of time for less cost. That is a goal worthy of pursuing. By growing cheaper food at a faster rate we all can obtain food like never before in the history of the world. The problem is that these food modifications aren't limited to the developing countries that need all the help they can get to have a stable food supply so they can begin to prosper. The problem is that almost *all* food today contains some form of this modification.

The backlash has begun against companies using these tactics to change the way food is raised. Organic food was an attempt to limit or prevent the use of pesticides and genetic and hormone modification in food. Sadly, the label "organic" is loose enough to allow many things into our food that the originators of the term do not want. But on the whole, organic produce is far healthier for you and your family than non-organic.

Note: Have you ever compared organic food to non-organic (called "conventional food") in the supermarkets that carry organic food? Often the organic food looks less healthy and goes old far faster once you get it home. Plus, it can be twice the cost. Who wants that? You should keep in mind a few things before forgoing the organic sections though because all is not always as it seems. First, food grown in a healthy environment is going to cost more. It also should *not* look better! Have you ever seen anything more beautiful than the perfect, beautiful apples as in the front bins of your grocery store? They are beautiful without blemish because the heavy pesticides kept every insect and animal away for acres and the wax used to polish those apples makes them look better than a freshly shined floor. Not having pesticides means that the organic produce might show a few signs of fatigue and perhaps initial bug attack here and there. Not having the cell-level modifications means they won't last as long as organic food because they haven't been laced with formaldehyde-like preservatives. They might only last as long as your great-grandparents' produce lasted. In other words, they are *normal, good-tasting, healthy food*. It's going to cost more if you want it. You can buy a cheap chair made from pressed particleboard or a more costly chair that will last far longer and be more comfortable. Everything is a choice.

The Organic Label Can Be a Concern Too

By the way, your great grandparents would not even be able to label their beef organic today. This is where some problems arise with such labeling. Organic beef means that the cattle never had antibiotics of any kind put in its system. But if your great grandfather's cow got an infection, your great grandfather would give the cow a shot of antibiotics and in 3 days the cow would be great. Such specific use of antibiotics is fine and is a long way from the antibiotic-laced food most cows are fed today from cradle to grave to ward off dying as baby calves since they are born, raised, and live in their own feces and fed genetically-engineered corn their whole lives. Cattle were designed to graze on grass in the fields and cows with that kind of life produce healthy milk and beef.

If you have a choice when it comes to your beef or chicken or pork, grass-fed and cage-free is actually preferred over pure organic. Smaller ranchers are beginning to understand this and are offering grass-fed beef and free-range chicks and pork. They avoid the term "organic" for their meats so they can get the animal well with antibiotics, when needed… which is rare. Otherwise, the animals roam the field while eating grass, bugs, and everything else they typical eat (chickens love bugs and those that can free-range during the daytime produce extremely healthy eggs and poultry meat for your family).

If it all seems complicated, it is. It didn't used to be.

One way to decide what kind of food is healthiest is to think back to this chapter's premise: your great grandparents ate far healthier than we do today. If you run across a farmer or rancher who raises crops and meat the way your great grandparents would have done it, you've found a wonderful supply of food for your family. Forget the labels organic and permaculture and high-brix and just use common sense when considering your food source.

Note: Use Google, if necessary, to find quality food locally.

Synergy – The Sum is Greater than the Individual Parts

Knowing all this helps your hormone levels in several ways. Your hormones need healthy and real food along with a few other commonsense things. They don't ask for much.

Sometimes exercise will boost a hormone. Sometimes a synthetic hormone is available when you cannot quite get enough help from food and exercise. (Sometimes synthetic hormones are bad too!) Sometimes a bio-identical hormone is available that is just like the hormones you produce at the cell level. Sometimes drugs will boost a needed hormone. Sometimes supplements will do so.

Our primary focus will be on the food you eat throughout the rest of this book. That is the very best way you can get your hormones into balance. That is also the very best way to feel your best and look your best. When supplements or a hormone replacement item has been found to be useful you'll read about it. In general though, food is going to be the prescription you use here to balance your key hormones.

Shortly we're going to cover a simple, easy-to-follow hormone-healthy diet. Then in the rest of this section, we change gears and focus on one hormone at a time. All of these hormones affect your health in major ways and ultimately are crucial for keeping your weight off forever.

It's the nature of a book like this to focus on one topic at a time, such as one hormone per chapter as the next several chapters do. Still, while you are focusing on individual hormones, keep in mind that *we* will stay focused on your overall health. We will always offer food advice that not only will boost a specific hormone but also will boost others, or at least the food will not negatively affect the other hormones along the way. We will stay holistic even when discussing individual hormones.

If you are out of balance in one or more hormones, only a good doctor, one who understands the importance of hormones and natural eating and supplementation, will be able to tell you for certain. Look in the phone book or on Google for local doctors who offer *chelation therapy.* Those who do often are in tune with proper nutrition and can test for key hormones through a series of full-spectrum blood and saliva tests. These doctors are less likely than a traditional and typical doctor who tries to treat symptoms first with drugs or surgery before they treat the root causes such as hormone imbalances through diet.

Note: Always get a full spectrum blood test that tests for as many of the key hormones as well as other health indicators such as sodium and potassium levels. If you accept a test that doesn't cover a full spectrum of hormones, you and your doctor are more likely to miss key connections between all your hormone levels that can help you zero-in on problems. Your physician must have knowledge of the way all your key hormones interact to properly evaluate any test results you get.

19

A HEALTHY HORMONE DIET

Is there a general eating plan that will help balance your hormones *and* help you lose weight dramatically *and* get you feeling great?

The simple answer is yes. This eating plan is not a diet. It is a lifelong style of eating that you and your family need to adopt.

Be warned: it takes guts because it goes against all that traditional advice of the past 40 years. It goes against what many of your grocery store signs and processed food boxes tell you. It goes against what most restaurants call "healthy" on menus. It goes against most diets you've ever heard of.

How can all those authority sources be wrong? A better question is this: How can hundreds of millions of great-grandparents who lived well into their 90s all be wrong? The simple answer is they were not wrong. They were healthy and did not suffer from the plethora of maladies that affect the general population today in spite of all our "medical advances." And they even ate lard almost every day. *Lard!*

Their diet should be your diet.

Hormonal Enemy #1: Sugar and Sugar Equivalents

Although we could go through every hormone and explain why sugar harms that hormone, it makes far more sense to cover it now in one spot.

The Most Wanted on the hormonal enemy list is sugar.

Name any sugar equivalent and it's just as dangerous: Honey, cane sugar, molasses, High Fructose Corn Syrup, fructose, dextrose, and virtually anything-*ose* actually.

"But didn't our great grandparents eat honey, molasses, fruit, and sugar?" you ask. That is a great question. Yes they did. They even spiked an iced tea with a spoonful of white sugar I bet. Maybe both at lunch *and* dinner!

But they didn't consume *22 teaspoons of sugar a day* and that is what the average American adult eats in one form or another. It gets worse. The average American teenager consumes *34 teaspoons of sugar each and every day* according to the American Heart Association.

That quantity of sugar is unnatural and our bodies simply don't know what to do with it all. The sugar is all around us in everything we eat. And it's worse now than ever. After the availability of low-fat and no-fat products have ballooned in every store. But the fat they removed, the fat that did not make us fat, tasted good. So they had to switch to something that tasted good. So they added a lot of sugar.

And over time the food companies, with the full approval of the governmental regulators who are supposed to oversee them instead of enable them, got wise to the fact that Americans realized sugar is deadly so they started putting other forms of sugar in our food to fool us. They called it something else. They used names that didn't have the word "sugar" in them. Like corn syrup. Cornstarch. Fructose. High Fructose Corn Syrup. Dextrose.

Note: High Fructose Corn Syrup is cornstarch boiled in acid. Its production is cheaper than normal, processed, white sugar but it is worse for you than sugar.

And over time, some Americans realized that all those non-"sugar" sugars still meant sugar so the food companies began reducing the amount of each one of those in our products for the few consumers who read the labels. You don't find one of those sugar equivalents in the first two or three ingredients any longer as much as you used to. But there are multiple *forms* of sugar throughout those ingredients, scattered here and there, so the total quantity of the sugar is still massive even though not one of the sugars gets top billing any longer in the ingredients.

Fooled us again, didn't they? And we keep getting fatter and unhealthier. And we keep getting sold more and more drugs to mask the symptoms that our sugar-laced food gives us.

It cannot be stressed enough: sugar kills. Yes, you can eat sugar in moderation. You know that is not what we're talking about here. We're not talking about moderation; we're talking about overdosing as almost every American does daily.

The number one way to feel better is to stop the sugar overdosing. *Now.* Don't plan to stop it next week. Stop it… *Now.* Don't plan to stop it after you finish the last piece of cake tonight for dessert. Stop it… *Now.*The number one way to begin aligning your hormones for health is to stop overdosing sugar… *Now.*

The "Good" Sugars: Honey, Molasses, Maple Syrup, Fruit, & Starches

Honey is sugar. Molasses is sugar. Maple syrup is sugar. Fruit is sugar.

If you get only organic honey, molasses, maple syrup, and fruit, guess what? They are all sugar also and the damage done is the same. Organic sugar isn't better for you than other sugar. It just isn't *quite* as deadly as the non-organic sugar.

Should you stop eating all those more natural sugar items? To play it safe, you should stop honey, molasses, maple syrup, and even fruit at least for a while until you can wean your body off sugar.

> **Note:** It turns out that both the 1-Day Diet *and* the 5:2 Diet (and the 10-Hour Coffee Diet) provide easy avenues for ridding sugar out of your diet while losing weight and improving your hormones! They are all win-win diets.

If you don't consider yourself a sugar, candy, or dessert person, there is still a huge chance you're addicted to sugar if you're an average American due to the amount of sugar you get elsewhere... like in bread and pasta. If you're not an American reading this, guess what? The reason your nation's thyroid problems, diabetes problems, cancer, and heart maladies have increased dramatically is that your nation isn't too far behind the USA in its injection of some form of sugar into virtually everything you eat.

Bread, corn, and potatoes are not sugar. However, starchy simple carbohydrates break down almost instantly into sugar as far as your body is concerned.

For most people reading this book, you need to be eating far less bread even if you don't eat desserts in traditional forms. Go *right now* and grab that loaf of bread on your counter, even if it's some fancy-named *High Heavy Multi-Grain Nut Stone-Milled* bread. Look at its ingredients. Go ahead, we'll wait here... Did you see it? The odds are great that your "healthy" bread has HFCS (High Fructose Corn Syrup). Look again if you didn't see it. It's rare that a loaf of bread sold today does not have HFCS.

Getting back to honey, every health food nut says honey is great for us, right? Honey is sugar. If sugar is bad, honey is bad.

Can honey help with allergies? Yes it can! If you can find an organic honey supplier within a few miles from your home, eating that honey may help your allergies and perhaps boost your immune system. Buying any other honey does not. And almost any honey sold on a supermarket shelf isn't even honey, but is Chinese-supplied substitute that looks and feels like honey... but is just a thick sugar slime.

If you find an organic honey supplier within a few miles of your home, keep that honey in your family's dietary mix. Half a teaspoon or perhaps a whole teaspoon every few days should be the limit. Anything more and the damage done by the honey's sugar wipes out any advantage done by the local honey.

You've heard that molasses is good for you, right? It can be! Organic black strap molasses is a great source of potassium. If you can find it (Amazon sells a good one here: http://

www.amazon.com/Organic-Blackstrap-Molasses-15-oz/dp/B000QV19BM/) then keep that molasses in your family's dietary mix. Half a teaspoon every few days. Just like the organic honey, anything more and the damage done by the molasses's sugar far offsets any advantage done by the organic black strap molasses.

You've heard that "real" maple syrup can be good for you, right? It can be! If you buy organic Grade B (never even *think* about buying Grade A ever again) Maple Syrup then you'll be getting the real thing, made the way nature intends you to eat it. (Amazon sells a good one here: http://www.amazon.com/Coombs-Family-Farms-Organic-32-Ounce/dp/B00271OPVU/.) Keep that organic Grade B maple syrup in your family's dietary mix. (Perhaps you can now predict what you're about to read next!) Half a teaspoon every few days. Anything more and the damage done by the Grade B maple syrup's sugar far offsets any health advantage done by the organic Grade B maple syrup.

Are you beginning to see a pattern?

By the way, why do you really need maple syrup? If you just love the taste then great, have it in the quantities described above. But if you need it for pancakes and waffles, guess what? As a general rule you should never in your life eat pancakes or waffles again. They are far worse than bread. And they are worse than fruit too. And you're about to see why fruit *can* be horrid.

Want your eyes opened in a way you never thought possible? Watch the following YouTube video about fructose, which is fruit sugar. It's called *Sugar: The Bitter Truth* and is here: http://www.youtube.com/watch?v=dBnniua6-oM&ob=av3e.

Remember those great-grandparents I keep talking about? You know, the ones who had healthy hormones all their lives? Yes, they ate fruit and perhaps a lot of it. They ate the fruit they grew. The fruit with its skin. When they had juice they would squeeze a couple of oranges or grapefruits once in a while into a glass and a lot of the pulp would fall into the glass too. Also, they'd have it with their morning meal. A meal full of eggs and bacon, often cooked in lard. *Lard!*

It turns out that the way fruit naturally occurs, with its skin is the way you should eat it. And it turns out that if you have a meal with lots of fat such as farm-raised, nitrite-free, nitrate-free, bacon made from pigs that led a happy life rooting up the field they were raised in, cooked in lard (*Lard!*) coming from those same happy pigs all slows down the negative effects of real fresh-squeezed fruit juice.

Note: Fat slows down your insulin secretions, which is one reason why whole milk causes you to gain less weight than skim milk. The fat slows down the milk sugar known as *lactose*.

Great-Granny ate fruit and drank her own fruit juice. If you can mimic the way she did it, by picking an apple off your own tree for instance, then go for it. But if your source of fruit is your grocer, even if organic, forget it. Eat no more than one serving of fruit daily if you're on a normal diet. Focus on berries, if possible.

How about the orange juice in the cans and cartons? You should eat an ice cream sundae instead. Because then you being honest with yourself. Then you will not be surprised when your hormones get all out of whack as they are going to anyway with all that orange juice over time.

Note: If you really want a sugar substitute, use Stevia and nothing else. Stevia is made from a plant and has zero effect on your glycemic index load. Just about all other artificial sweeteners make you crave sugar and elevate the acidity of your body's pH, which increases your chances to get sick. In addition, artificial sweeteners cause water retention and bloating.

Your Cells and Hormones Love Protein

Throughout the following that cover specific hormones you're going to see a lot of talk about eating more protein. Most hormones are made of protein. That is one reason why low-protein diets such as the Pritikin Diet are so dangerous to your hormonal balance. (The Pritikin Diet is also considered dangerous by many due to its strict limitation on fats.)

Note: Good protein never includes soy... or any ingredient that contains the word "soy" on the label anywhere.

Don't wait for an imbalance of hormones from a blood test. Just start eating more protein. *Now.* Eggs are perhaps the most perfect food in existence. They are literally *life building blocks*. Your hormones will benefit immediately from more eggs in your diet.[55]

And yes, you also need meat. Grass-fed beef, cage-free chicken, mercury-free fish, and free-rooting free-range locally grown pork.

Note: Nuts are a double-bonus for your hormones, body and weight because they provide both healthy fats and healthy proteins.

A Sidebar About Food

Living in the modern world exposes us to all sorts of toxins, both from industrial sites, products used in the building of homes and offices, aluminum from deodorants and old aluminum cookware (you should use an aluminum-free deodorant and only stainless steel and cast iron cookware without exception), mercury (from amalgam fillings and vaccinations and farm-raised fish), and plastics (if you like plastic containers, buy only BPA-free plastic), and municipal water supplies. It's good to be tested every few years or so to see if you need to detox from those and other toxins that stay in your cells.

We want to encourage you to begin eating only "real food" today.

Your great grandparents had it right by eating lots of eggs, butter, cooked in lard (*Lard!*),[56] chickens, cattle, bacon, vegetables they grew organically before "organic" was a garden-related word, and perhaps four teaspoons of sugar total daily from good fruit sources with the skin that they grew and an *occasional* sugar cube or honey scoop or maple syrup.

About Carbohydrates

You need carbs along with your good fats and proteins. Carbohydrates are not your enemy. Only some carbs are your enemy, especially in large quantities. Sugar, after all, is a carb. When eating carbs, try to limit your carb intake to about 20% to 25% of your daily food.

These suggested percentages are not fixed and you should not take them religiously. Worrying about your daily mix or fats/proteins/carbs can make you as crazy as counting calories and soon you'll just stop altogether if you fret too much with all the numbers.

But in general more fat and more protein and fewer carbohydrates than you eat now is what you should begin focusing on from this point forward. That means from now on, not during a "diet phase" but for a lifelong strategy for healthy hormones, healthy brains, and healthy bodies.

In general, as long as your carbohydrates are comprised of colorful vegetables, you can eat up!

Potatoes not only are starchy and have a high glycemic index that spikes your blood sugar and weight gain and hormone imbalance worse than scoop of ice cream (literally).[57] They also are root vegetables. They receive the bulk of pesticides sprayed on farms and gardens through runoff into the ground water where potatoes sit and grow.

You should eat green, leafy vegetables such as kale, lettuce (the greener the variety the better), spinach, okra, green beans, brown beans, all sorts of colorful peppers (even the hot ones, your metabolism gets a major boost every time!), squash, and tomatoes (technically tomatoes are fruit and amazingly they are *healthier* and more nutritious when cooked unlike most vegetables that should never be cooked too much if at all).

Stick to the green and colorful fibrous vegetables and you don't really need to concern yourself with a percentage of how much you eat. Just be sure that you have protein and fat at every meal. In general always eat your vegetables with protein and fat so you're not eating only carbs at any time.

If you like salads, do what the expensive restaurants do and cook slices of cage-free chicken to put over the salad and then sprinkle some walnuts and pecans on the salad. What a perfect combination! You'll get full from the salad, your short-term energy levels will be high due to the colorful veggies, and your long-term energy levels will remain high due to the chicken and nut proteins, and you won't feel full until it's truly time to eat next.

Grains Are Basically Bad

A little bread can be nice can't it?

"Our daily bread" is often a comfort food. By now you're no doubt convinced we're going to talk you out of buying most bread at most stores. True!

Know that, the best bread is bread that you or a friend makes from fresh, organic, ground wheat. You can get organic wheat to grind into bread in large "superpails" that stay good up to 15 years from Walton Feed.[58] Make sure you make "heavy" bread, bread with seeds and nuts in it. The grain will add fiber to your diet and the seeds and nuts will add to the taste and add protein and fat to the bread which slows down the negative effects of the bread's carbohydrate impact on your body.

Still, you don't want to over-eat this "good" bread. A slice or *maybe* two daily is the very outside maximum you should eat. Your body was not designed to handle many grains and you eat far too much bread right now if you're like the average person.

> **Note:** To help eliminate the negative effects of bread, you can add homemade or store-bought organic butter and extra virgin olive oil. To do as the Romans do, ground some organic, black pepper on top of all that oil and butter that you dribble all over the slice. The fat in the oil and butter does two things: makes the bread taste about as good as anything *can* taste and the bread will then have less impact on your blood sugar making the bread harder to show on your thighs! This is why a white, plain bagel clocks in at a higher glycemic load (meaning it impacts your blood sugar more and makes you fatter) than a scoop of premium ice cream! And low-fat yogurt almost doubles the glycemic load of that premium ice cream. Fat not only does *not* make you fat but it helps reduce the impact of food on your body. That's great because it tastes great and, for our purposes here, fat also is good for your hormones!

Stack Your Food Advantages

Driving through the Midwest you'll see miles and miles of corn fields. It's easy to forget that corn is not a vegetable but it's a grain. Like any grain, you want to limit corn in your family's diets. Your hormones react to corn about the same way they react to sugar because corn is a simple carbohydrate that becomes sugar quickly to your body.

Corn is worse than you might imagine. If you ever get a chance to see the documentary *King Corn* you should. You'll never eat the stuff again. What you may not know though is that corn is in everything you probably have eaten to this point. It's in almost every processed food. It's in almost every sugar equivalent. It's been in all the non-diet sodas the past couple of decades. (Diet soda is no better and is often worse with its aspartame and other chemical, phony sweeteners.)

> **Note:** You can get the movie *King Corn* here in DVD format: http://www.amazon.com/King-Corn-Standard-Packaging-Bledsoe/dp/B001EP8EOY/ ... even better, at the time of this writing, Amazon Prime members can watch the streaming version of *King Corn* for free here: http://www.amazon.com/King-Corn/dp/B003F9XQ9A/.

Corn is also in almost every bite of meat you eat!

From cradle to grave, most cattle, chickens and pigs are raised on a steady diet of corn. They are what they ate! This transfers to your body. Instead of grass for the cattle and bugs for the chickens and slop for the pigs they eat nothing... but... corn.

Then you get it second-hand. Like second-hand smoke, second-hand corn is bad for you and your hormones and your body. It's no longer "real" beef when the beef you eat was raised on a grain that its system was never designed to eat.

> **Note:** Fish farms feed fish a steady diet of soy. So when you eat most fish, especially any and all that comes in a package or canned, you're getting second-hand soy.

You probably already had more than your share of corn today second-hand. Until your diet consists of real food and real meat raised properly, avoid all corn.

Salt is Not Demonic

Salt is one of the most maligned foods of the past 50 years and is far less deadly than it's been blamed for in most people. Generally, someone who eats a diet rich in animal protein and healthy fats will not have a salt imbalance. Actually, you may find that you need to *add* salt to get enough of it. Let your cravings be your guide. But as you cease eating phony food from packages you will naturally get less salt and your body needs salt to perform well.

Still, a high craving for salt can result in a salt/potassium imbalance that does eventually cause you problems. A repaired serotonin level can help repair your salt craving and help return your sodium/potassium levels back to where they should be: in balance.

Some heart patients need to reduce salt. But salt is not bad for your heart in general and for a healthy society we need to look at some truth behind this condiment that is a required part of a healthy diet.

Like red meat, fat, and the sun, salt has gotten a tremendously bad rap. Your body needs an ample supply of sodium to function properly. When you begin to eat better you will eat fewer sugary or fast foods because your brain will want fewer of those kinds of things. Your sodium intake will go from a high amount of bad, processed, white salt to not enough salt.

Get salt and use it! Make sure, however, it is *sea salt*. Don't be afraid of it, especially as you eat higher quality foods that won't have as much sodium as the foods you used to binge on. I always carry either Celtic brand or Real Salt brand with me. Of the two, my preference is for the Real Salt brand. You can get it on Amazon.com here: http://www.amazon.com/Real-Salt-Sea-Pouch-26-Ounce/dp/B000BD0SDU/.

Sea salt is unprocessed (if you buy a good brand) and doesn't look uniformly white and is not as uniformly ground as the white, processed garbage you've seen. That is good and you should expect it. You will also find that it tastes much better than the typical salt. It's also much healthier for your body and hormonal balance than traditional table salt.

Sea salt has 84 different minerals whereas the typical table salt has only two.

More about that Sugar

Can you eliminate all non-fruit sweets from your life for a while? If there is any way you can do that you *will* stop craving sugar (hint: start with the 1-Day Diet). At first your body is going to go into minor withdrawals meaning you might crave sugar quite a bit and perhaps even feel shaky the first day or two depending on how much you eat now. That doesn't last long.

Our bodies secrete the hormone insulin to metabolize the food we eat. That is normal and that is what we want. The problem is that our bodies secrete insulin in much higher amounts when the foods are high in sugar or when our overall diets are high in bad carbs. Sugar damages your tissues so that your body tries to expel it from the bloodstream.

Higher insulin amounts make you feel hungrier and you end up eating more. That is why so many restaurants bring you a basket of bread before taking your order. That is also why Mexican restaurants bring you a basket of chips. That high-carb, low-fat, low-fiber bread and those chips spark your insulin secretion, lowers your body's ability to metabolize food, and makes you want to eat far more than you would have *before* filling up on bread.

Are you beginning to see the food-hormone connection?

Now for the Hormones

With the basic hormone-balancing diet out of the way, you need to focus now on specific hormones. By learning about the key hormones that affect your health and weight, you will learn to spot problems when they develop and learn ways to emphasize or use diet to augment specific hormones when an imbalance occurs.

20
THE MASTER CONTROL HORMONE

As with all the hormones we discuss, we're not out to make you a scientist. Hormones are a complex subject. But why complicate things? You want to be healthy and be at an optimum weight. That's our focus here.

It should be no surprise that your thyroid gland produces the thyroid hormone. The thyroid gland is located at the bottom of the front part of your neck.

Actually, there are two thyroid hormones: thyroxine and triiodothyronine.[59] Fortunately they are also referred to by the easier names of T4 and T3. T4 forms the bulk of your thyroid hormone group with the most active part being T3. We'll just call T4 and T3 the thyroid hormone and consider them as a pair to be a single group.

Your thyroid gland has a major job: it controls your metabolism (among other things including your energy levels). For someone interested in weight loss, therefore, getting the thyroid in balance is vital.

Problems with Thyroid Imbalance

"It's a glandular problem."

That is what people used to say about overweight people who couldn't seem to lose weight. It would often be said politely to help excuse the weight. It might be said sarcastically to mock the obese person. It may be said of the overweight person herself.

The thing is, being overweight *is* a glandular problem. Fortunately, it can be corrected in almost all cases. If you are overweight, it's almost a sure sign that your thyroid gland is not producing proper thyroid hormone levels.

Another sign of thyroid problems (or potential problems) is not just weight gain but swelling in the ankles and fingers. These are symptoms that portend to other problems such as low energy levels. It takes more energy to drag excess weight, and even swollen fingers and other body parts can make you sluggish.

Your fatigue from a thyroid imbalance adds to your weight gain in other ways too. With fatigue comes a false signal of hunger. This fatigue-related hunger signal usually makes you crave what is commonly called "comfort food." Traditionally comfort food is all the bad stuff: mashed potatoes, gravy, bread, corn, cake, and ice cream. By eating those heavy and bad carbs your thyroid goes into meltdown even further!

Chronic fatigue syndrome, a problem that was almost unheard of just a decade ago, has been on the rise. Thyroid imbalances cause that fatigue. This results in increased depression.

- Your thyroid also can produce non-metabolism related problems such as:
- Hair loss
- Dry and brittle hair and nails
- Extreme sensitivity to cold in your hands and feet
- Muscle and joint aches
- Low sex drive
- Menstrual cycle maladies
- Gastronomical problems such as constipation
- Lowered thinking ability

Thyroid issues have caused the drug industry to substantially boost its pills and liquids to treat the symptoms including an increased use of antidepressants, menstrual drugs, energy pills and drinks, pain relievers, sex drive boosters, laxatives, gelatin tablets, and so on.

Wouldn't it be easier and cheaper to treat the cause (the thyroid) and not all the symptoms? You can and the best news is that you often can treat the cause with diet alone.

Hypothyroidism

Fatigue-related thyroid problems are grouped together into a category known as *hypothyroidism*. Hypothyroidism is the result of an under-active thyroid that produces too few thyroid hormones.[60] Hypothyroidism, therefore, is a deficiency in thyroid hormones. You can exercise all day but you just won't lose weight or keep it off. Your body won't allow that. There is not enough thyroid activity to metabolize the fat.

Women are especially prone to hypothyroidism and get hypothyroidism almost ten-to-one over men. The most common age range is in the 40s where hypothyroidism flares up.

By moving less because you feel so tired, you don't get the daily benefit of normal caloric burning through movement as much as you would if you were more active.

Hyperthyroidism

Your thyroid doesn't just cause problems by being sluggish.

The opposite of hypothyroidism is *hyperthyroidism*. That is when your thyroid goes into hyper-activity. At first you might think hyperthyroidism is beneficial because if hypothyroidism makes you gain weight, then shouldn't we all strive for hyperthyroidism?

No, not at all.

We should all strive for a balanced thyroid. We want our thyroid hormone group to be at its optimum level the way they were designed to be.

The autoimmune disease known as *Graves Disease* is a type of hyperthyroidism. Fortunately, only a small number of people are susceptible to hyperthyroidism, around 2% for women and only about 0.2% of men. Excess sweating, hypersensitivity to heat, severe weight loss, and diarrhea can be present in hyperthyroidism's symptoms. You might note these are almost the mirror image of hypothyroidism's symptoms of being cold all the time, weight gain, and constipation.

You want neither hyperthyroidism not hypothyroidism.

Putting Your Thyroid in Balance

Those with thyroid problems have several non-medical tips to try and many people see good results without going the drug route.

First, iodine supplementation is often suggested as a means to bring your thyroid into balance. Next to a deficiency in vitamin D3, nutritionists are beginning to suspect that a lack of iodine in our diets contributes to problems never-before seen in the numbers we see them today. Decades and decades ago the RDA (*recommended daily allowance*) of nutrients was designed and has hardly been updated since.

So our RDA of nutrients such as iodine has not increased but the problem is that the food we eat *has* decreased in the nutrients we get from it. So whereas out great grandparents might have done well on a "normal" diet back then, today's "normal" is anything but normal when it comes to healthy bodies and balanced hormone. The RDA for iodine has been said to be off as much as an *entire decimal place*, meaning instead of the 10 or so mcg (micrograms) suggested, we need as much as 10 to 15 mgs (milligrams) daily… about 100 times the RDA's suggested level.

A blood test can tell you immediately how your thyroid health is doing. But if your thyroid is out of balance, certainly you owe it to yourself to try some iodine supplementation and better food before you go the thyroid medicine route. Let your nutritionist determine from your blood test what levels of iodine you should supplement with, if any. Excess levels of iodine are just as bad as low levels. Excess iodine blocks the enzymes that produce thyroid hormones.

You might think you get ample supplies of iodine in salt. It's true that salt *can* be beneficial to your thyroids health. Still, salt as it is generally eaten is not good for you. It is processed and the iodine is a mass-produced substance that, like most "enriched" food and condiments, has better alternatives. Instead of the perfectly symmetrical table salt, start using only sea salt as discussed earlier. Sea salt does have traces of iodine, but a blood test will tell you if you might need an extra boost in iodine. If so, *Idoral*, a potassium and iodine supplement, is available here: http://www.amazon.com/Iodoral-Potency-Potassium-Supplement-Tablets/dp/B000WG3FU4/.

Idoral is a non-prescription supplement and it's great. But as you know, when you can fix or begin to repair any malady with real food, that's always the best alternative. Our problem is that we usually create problems by not eating real food. Polyunsaturated oils like soybean and corn oil block absorption of the iodine needed to make proper levels of the thyroid hormone.

One way to help hypothyroidism is with Brazil nuts. Brazil nuts are high in selenium and selenium helps regulate your thyroid hormones.

In addition to Brazil nuts, the entire hormone-balanced dietary lifestyle discussed earlier is almost a perfect food-based prescription for good thyroid balance. All the good fats, the seeds, nuts, and oils, all contribute to help balance your thyroid hormones. (Thyroids especially like cod liver oil, even if we don't. Fortunately, cod liver oil is now sold in easy-to-take capsules, such as here: http://www.amazon.com/Barleans-Organic-Oils-Softgels-250-Count/dp/B0031ESWZW/)

Quality sourced beef, lamb, and mercury-free fish such as wild Alaskan salmon are great for your thyroid. Vegetables and small amounts of fruit also contribute to thyroid health.

It's been found that snacking between meals not only affects your weight gain but also eating more frequently slows down your thyroid function. Stick to "three square" meals a day if you're not doing the 1-Day Diet, 5:2 Diet, or the 10-Hour Coffee Diet. Stay away from sodas; especially diet sodas. Just about any "low-fat" or "no-fat" food labeled as such is phony food that will not help your thyroid at all.

So the next time you sit down to eat a meal, make every bite count and stack all your advantages. Eating a high fat, high protein, low carb, healthy meal with organic produce is going to rev up your master control hormone into superhero gear.

21
THE FAT-STORING HORMONE

Insulin is a hormone produced by your pancreas.

The pancreas shares some space with your stomach by resting right behind it.[61] Its location is perfect because insulin produced by your pancreas gland goes into action when food is present in your system. The type of food you eat determines how much insulin your pancreas produces.

Insulin determines the way our body uses or stores food. Insulin's role is to regulate the metabolism of these two food groups:

Fat

Carbohydrates

Diabetes problems have been on the rise ever since the government told everybody how much healthier it is to eat fewer fats and more carbohydrates. Insulin problems are diabetes problems. How important is insulin? People who live long lives have normal insulin levels.

A Little Insulin Background

To discuss insulin properly, we must get into the chemical behavior of insulin just a bit more than most of the other hormones.

As we eat carbohydrates, our bodies convert those carbs into sugar, which secretes into our bloodstream from our intestines. This is normal and proper. What is improper is when our sugar levels get out of balance, which happens as we eat more sugar and fewer fats and proteins.

Sugar, in the form of glucose, is what travels from our intestines to our blood supply. Too much glucose sugar and we die because an abundance of glucose is toxic. Our pancreas creates insulin to regulate the amount of glucose in our system. Glucose levels rise while we eat carbs, our pancreas creates more insulin and the insulin is the signal to our liver and muscles and fat tissue to remove glucose from our bloodstream. That removed glucose converts to glycogen and is stored in our cells.

The more sugar our food has, the more that glucose rises. Excess insulin causes excess glucose to be removed. As long as everything is in balance, all is well. We can even eat a sweet orange and the pancreas generates insulin to remove the excess glucose from our blood. The excess glucose can get stored as glycogen.

If we haven't eaten for a while, or if we eat non-sugary foods, our blood glucose levels fall below normal. That is when our bodies begin to use its stored glycogen as energy. The upshot is that we lose some weight every time stored glycogen is used for fuel instead of glucose.

So, although we use sugar for fuel, sugar is damaging to our cell tissues, which is why a healthy body performs a constant give-and-take with insulin. A healthy body with a healthy diet works to use carbohydrates for fuel and not for storing fat in cells.

Type 1 Diabetes

Things happen where we don't always produce enough insulin when it's needed.

People with type 1 diabetes don't produce enough insulin. Their bodies enter into a starvation cycle even when they eat because their cells don't utilize the calories from the glucose they pull from their bloodstream. The patients get sick if they don't get regular insulin injections to allow the cells to utilize the glucose properly.

Type 2 Diabetes

Type 2 diabetes is about 9.5 times more common than type 1 diabetes.

Whereas type 1 diabetes patients don't create enough insulin, type 2 diabetes patients often produce too much insulin and the body becomes insulin resistant. The cells ignore insulin signals and don't pull glucose from the bloodstream. Too much glucose in the blood is toxic and type 2 diabetes patients get sick from the high levels of glucose in their blood.

In the past, type 2 diabetes occurred generally in patients in their 40s and older. It even had the label, "adult onset diabetes" that hasn't been used lately due to the new prevalence of the disease in children. Type 2 diabetes often results from being overweight.

My 1 Day Diet actually helps to reverse and correct type 2 diabetes by making your body more insulin sensitive. If want to lose weight as fast as possible from a diet *and* have type 2 diabetes, do yourself a favor and try the diet immediately.

Putting Your Insulin in Balance

Obviously, if you're diagnosed with diabetes, seek medical help.

Although we're convinced that our bodies are designed to utilize real food to regulate and repair our systems, if we get too far out of balance we require medical help. Not enough time is available to wait on our bodies to fix things if the damage has gone too far.

Note: Insulin affects the production of other hormones including glucagon, leptin, cortisol, testosterone, and estrogen. This is yet another reason to focus on your insulin balance.

For example, if you're diagnosed with type 1 diabetes you must be treated with insulin, either through injections or pumps. Your body requires the insulin for properly digesting all the food you eat. If you're diagnosed with type 2 diabetes, you may be put on medicine, depending on the severity, but your doctor is going to give you the same advice we will: your diet will have a dramatic impact on how much your type 2 diabetes is a problem in your life.

If your doctor recommends a high carb diet, you'd better get a second opinion. Neither Jen nor Rich are doctors and we don't play one in the books we write. Nevertheless, the more carbs you eat the higher your blood sugar levels will spike.

Alcohol, starchy foods, and desserts contribute to insulin problems. Just about anything that comes in a box at your grocery store is either a dead food that is neutral or a substance that is going to affect your insulin hormones negatively.

The Role that Exercise Plays

A sedentary lifestyle without exercise can also raise diabetes complications. You don't have to become an exercise guru to escape a sedentary lifestyle. Just get up every hour and walk around if nothing else! Your body is designed for regular activity and that activity doesn't have to be extreme.

Don't try to set exercise time records!

One thing to avoid if you want balanced hormones is extended exercise over weeks and months. When you exercise using a paced, high-intensity followed by low-intensity pattern your hormones are made healthier and more plentiful when needed. If, however, you are a marathon kind of runner, swimmer, aerobic-related exerciser or you lift weights using set after set 5 days a week or more, your hormones are so busy trying to repair damage done by the exercising that they don't get enough time to regulate your digestive activities.

According to Eric Berg, DC, fat-burning hormones do their best work during resting activities and not exercising activities, but the exercising is vital to benefit from the recovery periods.[62] Give your body plenty of time to rest and recover from the exercise you choose.

Exercise lowers your insulin levels (and increases glucagons, which is win-win for you!). Some diabetes patients monitor their blood sugar levels close to bedtime and if they are too high they must walk on a treadmill or do other forms of exercise until their blood sugar level is low enough to go to sleep safely. Why not get started before you have to lower your blood sugar level before bed every night on a treadmill?

Don't *plan* to start exercising, just *start* exercising.

If you have not exercised in a long time just walk in place while you watch television tonight instead of just sitting or lying there. Getting started is the hardest part, so stop *planning* to start and just start. And again, don't believe the aerobics lie that long exercise sessions, such as long-distance running, are healthy. That kind of exercise creates more dangerous free radicals in your body and causes numerous hormonal imbalances over the long term.

Exercise in short, explosive bursts… you'll be challenging your body with what it needs most.

Back to Food

MSG often found in Asian food and many other items has been shown to *triple* the output of insulin that you produce. Try to avoid any and all Asian food places that don't state they are MSG free.

The supplement called *chromium picolinate* can be an important help for blood sugar regulation. Start with 3,000 mcg (*micro*grams) daily to begin with and reduce that down to 1,000 mcg daily after your sugar cravings go away.

22
THE FAT-REMOVING AND
THE "I FEEL FULL" HORMONES

Like insulin, glucagon is a hormone that your pancreas produces.

Glucagon raises low blood sugar when needed. When your blood sugar level gets too low, a healthy pancreas releases glucagon. Glucagon has been called a fat burning or removing hormone.[63]

You'll recall from the previous chapter that when blood sugar levels get too high, a healthy pancreas releases insulin to remove the glucose from your blood and send that glucose to your other tissue. Isn't the body's regulation system amazing? It's worth balancing your hormones and keeping them balanced because they keep you feeling good through their behind-the-scenes activities such as blood-sugar level regulation.

The bottom line of glucagon is that it melts fat. When your blood sugar levels are low, you'll secrete glucagon so your tissues get needed sugar and energy. Glucagon pulls sugar out of storage, first from the liver, then from fat.

Problems with Glucagon Imbalance

If you have little glucagon, you'll become fat. If you have too much glucagon, you'll be thinner than you should be.

Although most people dream of being thinner than they should be, such a problem can be as dangerous as obesity. Remember that a healthy hormonal balance will not only enable you to lose weight if you're obese but a healthy hormonal balance will add weight if you need that. Your body knows what weight is best for you as long as you focus on your hormones and let them regulate your weight the way they were designed to do.

The way you mess up your glucagon balance is to eat too many bad foods over a long period of time. This is what so many are doing right now. Snacking between meals with a quick candy bar or soda pop also damages glucagon levels.

Note: Pancreatic tumors can be present which almost certainly will lead to out-of-balance glucagon levels so if you have had trouble with weight loss in the past you should have your pancreas checked to make sure it's clear.

If you get hungry between meals, eat some organic, mixed nuts. 10 to 20 grams of protein also prevents your body from entering a starvation stage if you go too long without eating. If that happens, your body will begin to crave bad carbs dramatically. Also, your body will try to hang on to fat stores in case the perceived fast lasts a while.

Putting Your Glucagon in Balance

When glucagon metabolizes your fat into energy, you lose weight.

Eat natural fats and a good amount of protein while avoiding bad carbs, your insulin secretion is regulated. This also will mean your glucagon is regulated and in order. Protein is instrumental in stimulating glucagon.

Exercise also increases glucagon production. You already know that exercise burns fat. But now you know that exercise produces a fat-burning hormone that burns even more fat!

The "I Feel-Full" Hormone

Leptin is a hormone that controls how full you feel. With no other description you already can see how vital controlling leptin is if you want to control your weight.

Unlike many other hormones, no gland secretes leptin. Your fat cells secrete leptin.

Problems with Leptin Imbalance

Leptin can be a strange hormone in how it gets out of balance.

If you eat too little food you can develop low leptin levels. One problem of calorie-restriction diets – and there are several problems with calorie-restriction diets – is that leptin is reduced.

In women, menstruation can slow and even stop if leptin hormone levels get too low.

Strict low-carb diets with a restrictive level of all carbohydrates can cause your body to produce too little leptin. The Atkins diet suggests only a few weeks of the "induction phase" which is good because reducing carbs down to 10% or so can drop your leptin levels. This is one reason why some people see how well low-carb diets work and they go overboard without eating enough carbs to maximize their weight loss. In doing so, they damage their leptin levels causing other problems to appear.

Leptin increases when you eat too many fake, processed foods. You keep eating but your satiety goes into overload and the full switch breaks and you lose control of your appetite. In other words, you keep eating more and more but you never feel full. Leptin levels stop responding properly.

In general, the more you weigh the more leptin you produce. But instead of working for you, the leptin hormone begins working against you. When you are overweight, your leptin hormone level increases but at the same time, that obesity causes those leptin hormones to become sluggish and misfire. In spite of the quantities, they stop turning off your "full" switch. You therefore eat more and more which contributes to the obesity cycle you find yourself on.

> **Note:** Low-fat diets are bad for at least two primary hormones. They lead to both high insulin and high leptin levels.

An article about Dr. Kent Holtorf, MD recently said this in an interview where he linked leptin and thyroid (T3) as key factors in the inability to lose weight:[64]

Dr. Holtorf has discovered that while there are many factors involved in the inability to lose weight, almost all the overweight and obese patients he treats have demonstrable metabolic and endocrinological dysfunctions that contribute to weight challenges. In particular, Dr. Holtorf addresses the evaluation and correction of imbalances in two key hormones – leptin and reverse T3 (rT3) – to help thyroid patients lose weight.

Studies are finding [...] that the majority of overweight individuals who are having difficulty losing weight have varying degrees of leptin resistance, where leptin has a diminished ability to affect the hypothalamus and regulate metabolism. This leptin resistance results in the hypothalamus sensing starvation, so multiple mechanisms are activated to increase fat stores, as the body tries to reverse the perceived state of starvation.

The mechanisms that are activated include diminished TSH secretion, a suppressed T4 to T3 conversion, an increase in reverse T3, an increase in appetite, an increase in insulin resistance and an inhibition of lipolysis (fat breakdown).

These mechanisms may be in part due to a down-regulation of leptin receptors that occurs with a prolonged increase in leptin.

The result? Once you are overweight for an extended period of time, it becomes increasingly difficult to lose weight.

That last sentence is key because it means the longer you go without correcting your leptin and other hormonal balance issues, the harder it is going to be to lose weight.

Putting Your Leptin in Balance

To lose weight as quickly as you can you *must* get your leptin into balance.

Healthy fats are crucial for proper leptin balancing. You must maintain your good fats, making them a major part of your lifestyle for the rest of your life. In doing so, you will feel full after eating a good meal and you will feel hungry when you need to eat.

It is your fat that produces leptin. Leptin, when in balance, tells your brain's hypothalamus that you are full and can stop eating.

Note: Healthy fats and fish contain high levels of something called omega-3 oils, which are generally in short supply in the modern, fast food lifestyle. Among other advantages, omega-3 oils boost your feeling of being full after eating and help regulate healthy levels of leptin.

Sleep is critical for proper leptin levels. This means that your sleep hormone – melatonin – also comes into play, indirectly, to regulate leptin.

In addition to healthy fats and more sleep, low leptin levels have been helped by the supplement 5-HTP. 5-HTP, also known as *5-Hydroxytryptophan*, is a by-product of the protein building block called L-tryptophan. You can find a quality 5-HTP supplement here: http://www.bodybuilding.com/store/now/5htp.html.

23
THE GROWING UP HEALTHY HORMONE

When little children grow up, they get bigger. They get bigger because they secrete GH – the *growth hormone*.

This GH growth hormone is secreted naturally in your body by your pituitary gland. HGH, or human growth hormone, is created by a fancy technology called *recombinant DNA technology*. In spite of those technical differences most sources, including this one, will refer to HGH and GH interchangeably because the mainstream does so. Unless specifically mentioning a lab-produced growth hormone in which case we'll always stick to the more specific HGH.

HGH affects growth and repair of all your muscles and tissues. The reason the growth hormone can repair your tissues is that it has responsibility for helping to reproduce cells throughout your body. Every one of your body's cells is replaced multiple times as you age. The "you" you started with isn't the same "you" now reading this book!

Therefore you maintain this proper rebuilding of your cells you must maintain a proper level of GH production. You must also maintain a proper weight. Body fat inhibits your production of HGH secretion. If you are overweight then your body is doing everything it can to produce HGH and almost certainly failing.

Problems with HGH Imbalance

The time your body needs high doses of growth hormone is your formative younger years of course. You are growing up and that's why it's called the *growth* hormone. Too much

HGH as a child is a rare disorder but can appear once in a while manifesting itself as extra-large (not necessarily overweight) children. Too much as an adult is rare and found mostly in athletes who abuse growth hormone supplements.

As you age, you naturally will produce less HGH. As long as you're otherwise healthy, that is fine and even medical doctors don't prescribe the HGH therapies for patients who are otherwise healthy. So a decrease related to aging is not a major problem. You slow down as you age, your metabolism slows, you eat less, you are less active, your body is expected to do less, so less HGH is often not noticed or a problem. If anything, less growth hormone in an elderly person means that person won't have an over-abundance of HGH, which although rare, can lead to enlargement of bones and breast tissue in men.

Having too little HGH too early is far more common. Children who are far smaller and weaker than other children their age possibly have HGH development problems. Of course diets that make our children fat and diabetic – the government's Food Pyramid-related diets – will put HGH and many other hormones out of balance long before these children have a chance to reach adulthood in a healthy state.

- Adults with low HGH production experience several seemingly unrelated symptoms including:
- Sleep without dreams (routine dreaming is a healthy release for a healthy brain)
- Reduction in overall muscle mass
- Fatigue
- Anxiety
- Lack of sexual interest
- Panic

Sadly, many people and doctors see symptoms such as these and look to psychology and psychiatry to handle them. Out of ignorance and perhaps greed, those fields rarely will do anything to address the hormonal balance issues so many people have today.

Ways to Put Growth Hormone Out of Balance

One way that HGH is kept from being freely produced in your body is through frequent eating. You might be noticing a trend here because other hormones such as thyroid production of insulin and glucagons, are also negatively affected by frequent eating.

Typically, a weight-loss book will stress that you should eat smaller meals more frequently instead of three large daily. The problem is that this does your hormones no favor. If your hormones become too stressed out working on your digestion functions they won't be putting enough effort into producing balanced hormones. So in general, eating two to three meals daily is one healthy way to benefit your hormones. When your hormone levels benefit your weight will too.

Note: HGH levels increase when you fast, but fasting is tricky. Performing a starvation fast for example can wreak havoc with your whole body depending on your condition before you began and how to approach the starvation fast. In addition, starvation fasts are difficult and unnecessary with the good alternatives available if weight is a key goal for you. Fortunately, the 1-Day Diet and 10-Hour Coffee Diet solve all this fasting mystery for you and is the best diet for weight loss and long-term health.

At the time of this writing, growth hormones cannot be added to cows for beef production or to chickens or pigs. It is still legal to put growth hormones in dairy cows, however, to increase their production of milk.

Alcohol can decrease HGH levels. Remember that alcohol is basically sugar. You've heard that some red wine can add a life-extending substance called *resveratrol* to your system. But keep in mind that alcohol is sugar and sugar is basically toxic to your system which is why you might get drunk on a little bit of whiskey but not on the same amount of water or iced tea.

Perhaps you're tired of sugar being to blame for so many problems in this book. We are too! We wish that a 2 liter cola and a Snickers bar were healthy foods!

Actually, we've been eating so well for so long that just thinking about both of those make us sort of queasy to our stomachs. That's the good news about eating properly. Your body automatically turns on rejection mechanisms to keep you away from the bad stuff. It takes months of eating badly to wear down your rejection mechanisms and to make your hormone response so sluggish that you no longer reject those phony food items and begin to crave them. A broken body and a broken hormone balance craves sugar because the hormones are not able to sync up well enough to give you a genuine feel-good feeling so you seek outside sources than only make the problems worse.

But if for no other reason, you must get off the sugar bandwagon to look better. Yes, a piece of frozen pie from your grocer's freezer is not going to cause you long-term problems by itself.

Putting Your HGH in Balance

The formula that begins putting your HGH in balance *and keeping it there* is extremely similar to other hormones. That's the whole beauty of approaching your hormone balancing act yourself, at least before you seek medical help other than to get initial testing to see if any of your hormones are out of whack. That beauty is that hormones seem to respond negatively to many of the same things and hormone balance seems to prefer many of the same things across the whole spectrum of hormones.

You know the dietary route well by now. It's just what you expect because your body is not crazy. What is good for your body in one place is almost always good for the rest of your body. Protein seems to be more important even than fat for good HGH secretion so don't let your protein intake drop. Eat good protein at every meal.

Note: The fast food chain named *Chipotle* is known for its hormone-free ingredients and its grass-fed beef, pork, and cage-free chickens. Chipotle attempts to source some of its food locally throughout the United States close to the restaurant locations that use the food. They are not 100% grass-fed and cage-free but they are working towards that goal and should be commended. The movie *Food, Inc.,* is an excellent documentary showing you the poor health of the nation's FDA- and USDA-approved food supply. One of the extra features on the disc is a segment about Chipotle's food sourcing that is eye opening. It'll make you want to load up your family tonight and take them there! Not only will your family like the taste, so will your hormones! (Go easy on the rice.)

Routine exercise also improves your HGH production. You don't have to become a fitness guru; actually, doing too much seems to cause your hormones to react badly. But move around, go outdoors on breaks and get some sun, swim, play recreational sports with your family, and just have a moderately active lifestyle to stave off many aches, pains, and hormonal maladies that can arise faster from a sedimentary lifestyle.

Since you're going to eat better and move around more, your HGH will be happier and more productive. In addition, other hormone levels will spike to good levels and you'll sleep better too. It turns out that good sleep habits also improve HGH levels.

It's like your body's internal parts are designed to work together in a system!

Supplementing with HGH

Lots of problems arise with HGH drug supplementation. In general, there is a good reason why even medical doctors refuse to give HGH to otherwise healthy patients who request it.

24
UP AND DOWNS: THE SLEEP AND STRESS HORMONES

Next to insulin, melatonin is one of the most widely known hormones.[65]

International travelers take melatonin while crossing multiple time zones in an attempt to get their sleep pattern modified for the upcoming night. Insomnia sufferers have melatonin supplements in their bathroom cabinets.

Unlike many other hormones such as HGH, melatonin supplements are available over-the-counter and when used at their intended doses provide virtually no side effects. If nothing else, hopefully the prevalence of melatonin has reduced the usage of Ambien and its reported psychedelic side effects that lead to additional problems.

Having said that, people do pop melatonin without much thought to its intended use and it's best to approach anything like that with some knowledge.

So here is some knowledge.

How Melatonin Cycles You Up and Down

Throughout the day, your levels of melatonin secretion rise and fall. The reason is that melatonin levels change is that our activity levels change. In the optimum state, melatonin levels increase at night when we sleep and decrease during the day to keep us active. If our schedules change, such as we begin working the night-shift or switch time zones due to travel, out cycles can get out of alignment for a while until our bodies realize that they need to modify the release cycle of melatonin.

Melatonin is an antioxidant to help ward off dangerous oxidizing agents in bodies and food. As with metal that gets rusty after it comes out of water and hits oxygen, oxygen can damage your body through a normal process that a healthy diet and good levels or hormones such as melatonin inhibit. "Free radicals" form from oxidation, which attack our systems if not kept under routine check by the rest of our body.

As you age, you normally sleep less because melatonin production is reduced through the normal process of aging. Teenagers who insist on staying up late and sleeping late aren't *fully* to blame for their insistence on such a schedule because in the teen years melatonin production appears a little later at night and produces longer into the early morning hours than at other times in our lives.

There is evidence that melatonin helps protect against immunity disorders, although the research is still being finalized and verified across the world.

Problems with Melatonin Imbalance

Besides a bad night's sleep, too little melatonin can result in an under-production of a hormone called cortisol, which you'll learn about in the next chapter. (Cortisol and melatonin, when not in balance, are somewhat enemies and can work against each other.)

Having to sleep in the daytime hours or having to stay awake at night after dark is more difficult due to the fact that light and darkness trigger melatonin decreases and increases. We truly are made to sleep at night when it's dark and be awake in the day when it's light.

Low melatonin has been linked to autism and premature aging. Although a lack of melatonin has not been said to be a cause, melatonin supplementation is sometimes helpful for those who suffer from migraines and cluster headaches.

Too much melatonin is rare and even when supplementation is too much, the side effects have not been recorded as major at this time.

Putting Your Melatonin in Balance

Often what fixes a good night's sleep helps your melatonin production. When you sleep, even if work forces you to be a day sleeper, you want the room as dark as possible to get your body secreting melatonin. Even digital clocks and the television in an otherwise dark room can impair your melatonin production.

As stated earlier in this book, a good night's sleep not only makes you healthier, wealthier, and wise (actually, it may have been Ben Franklin who said that...), a good night's sleep has also been found to aid in weight loss. You know you feel better when you've slept well and you think better and feel better on the whole.

If you need additional help to sleep better, using a 3mg melatonin supplement such as the one found here helps for short-term sleeping problems and time-zone adjustments: http://www.amazon.com/Foods-Melatonin-High-Grade-Capsules/dp/B0019LTGC2/

Depending on your weight and muscle mass, up to 9mg might be necessary to achieve optimal sleep. You may have to play around with the dosage a while to see what works well for you. Don't immediately jump to 9mg if you haven't tried melatonin before, however, because taking more when you don't need it can actually inhibit your sleep cycle.

Some people see better results with liquid drops instead of the tablets. You can get 2.5mg drops here:

http://www.amazon.com/Natrol-Melatonin-2-5-Liquid-8-Ounce/dp/B001HCOFMO/

Note: When using drops, it's suggested that you put the drop or drops under your tongue for a few seconds instead of swallowing it directly. This can raise the effectiveness of the drops by getting the melatonin into your blood supply more quickly than swallowing the melatonin.

The Stress Hormone

Your adrenal glands produce the hormone called cortisol. With adrenal problems you're often tired and down during the day and you cannot sleep at night. An adrenal hormone deficiency can give you strong cravings for chocolate. This is because your body's serotonin (the feel-good chemical in your brain) is created by the adrenal glands. Chocolate stimulates serotonin. People who crave chocolate are actually craving serotonin.

When you have anxiety, fear, or other forms of stress your body secretes more cortisol. Cortisol enables you to better handle stress. But cortisol also works with your metabolism-related system. Cortisol raises your blood sugar level when it gets too low. Your energy level is directly affected by how well balanced your cortisol level is.

Problems with Cortisol Imbalance

As you'll see later, a prolonged cortisol rise can work against other hormones, especially DHEA, that help offset the effects of too much cortisol. Cortisol can begin to cause damage when left unchecked.[66]

If your body produces too much cortisol, for example, then your melatonin is reduced. The excess cortisol doesn't allow your melatonin secretions to occur naturally. Your sleep therefore becomes more difficult. Other problems soon can follow such as extended insomnia and depression.

The "happy" brain chemical called *serotonin*[67] shuts down with too much cortisol production. Your mood will be depressed and your interest in life's normal activities can drop. Sexual problems can arise, especially lack of desire. The combination of little sleep and slower response, results in weight gain, especially around your stomach.

A lack of cortisol production, which is less common than excess cortisol, results in diarrhea, which works with other factors to cause unnatural and rapid weight loss.

Out-of-balance cortisol levels can result in major diseases such as Cushing's Disease and diabetes. Cosmetically, dark circles under your eyes can appear demonstrating high cortisol levels. (Such dark circles might also be a result of HGH deficiency too.)

If you have weight gain and cannot seem to lose fat, or you have a lack of interest in daily activities and have little interest in sex, get your cortisol levels checked.

Putting Your Cortisol in Balance

Sugar is a danger for cortisol imbalanced patients. You need to avoid sugar in all forms (we sound like a broken record, but we need to keep saying it) including alcohol to try to get your cortisol levels back into their normal range. High cortisol levels are more common in people who eat fast foods and processed and pre-packaged foods because excess salt can also damage cortisol levels.

If you're eating correctly and eating a hormone-healthy lifestyle you almost certainly don't get too much salt and that sodium shouldn't be a problem even if you add it to some of your meals once in a while.

Exercise alone doesn't necessarily improve cortisol, but exercise does help you deal with stress better, so exercise can reduce stress in your body and mind and keep cortisol functioning more normally.

Whatever you do get some good fats into your diet. Low-fat diets can negatively affect your cortisol levels.

Eat regularly and don't skip meals. Doing so can cause your body to literally cannibalize itself by taking muscle tissue from your leg area to be converted to glucose-based sugar fuel for energy. (Obviously, doing the 1-Day Diet as outlined in not a concern in regards to skipping meals and eating regularly.)

25
THE HUNGER-STIMULATING AND REBUILDING HORMONES

Your stomach and pancreas secrete ghrelin… a hormone that stimulates your appetite.

In a way, ghrelin prepares you for meals because before you eat, your ghrelin increases and when you finish – if properly secreted – your ghrelin levels decrease. If you go too long without eating, your ghrelin level will rise accordingly in an effort to get you to look for food.

Actually, when you just *think* of food your ghrelin will increase in an effort to prepare you for a potential meal. Unlike leptin, which rises to make you feel satisfied after eating, a rising level of ghrelin makes you feel hungry.

When you're hungry, you typically are not depressed. Hunger is a motivator to find food and not a depressant. Therefore, indirectly ghrelin acts as a natural anti-depressant.

Problems with Ghrelin Imbalance

One reason why lack of sleep can increase your weight gain is because serotonin is a brain chemical that naturally flattens your production of ghrelin when ghrelin is unneeded. Without the controlling serotonin, your ghrelin stays high and you stay hungry. Fortunately, a hormone-healthy diet such as the 1-Day Diet (or the 5:2 Diet) is brain healthy and can help maintain a proper level of serotonin too.

So, when you can increase your level of serotonin you get more sleep. More sleep causes your ghrelin levels to rise. The elevated ghrelin levels do two things:

1. Boosts your HGH

2. Reduces your cravings for carbohydrates, enabling you to eat better food with higher good fats and proteins.

To help clarify what high ghrelin can do, ScienceDaily.com, one of the most popular science news websites, described an in-depth study of sleep and ghrelin funded by the National Institute of Health. ScienceDaily.com said the following in their October 4, 2010 edition:

Higher ghrelin levels have been shown to "reduce energy expenditure, stimulate hunger and food intake, promote retention of fat, and increase hepatic glucose production to support the availability of fuel to glucose dependent tissues," the authors note. "In our experiment, sleep restriction was accompanied by a similar pattern of increased hunger and … reduced oxidation of fat."

Putting Your Ghrelin in Balance

Get a restful night's sleep by supplementing with melatonin if you need to. This boosts your serotonin and keeps your ghrelin in check so that your ghrelin appears when you need to eat but then goes away. Like nosy neighbors, the hormone ghrelin is something you don't want to stick around too long after a meal.

Obviously a hormone-healthy lifestyle of eating will help ghrelin and the hormones connected with ghrelin. Everything in your body seeks to be in balance because all the parts work together to keep you alive. It's in your best interest to help your hormones. Plus you'll feel so much better and lose weight.

Note: A new vaccine is being tested that is called the *anti-obesity vaccine*. We're not too fond of this "solution" to weight loss but it's interesting to look at while discussing ghrelin. This vaccine uses your own body's immune system to suppress the production of ghrelin. This suppresses your appetite. Now with vaccines come costs: they are a non-food answer, and known sometimes to add toxic mercury to your system and such an anti-obesity vaccine working to suppress a normal and needed hormone seems like something to be avoided. Only time will tell whether or not the anti-obesity vaccine lives up to its name or not. Extremely obese patients may very well need extra help to lose initial weight. The problem comes if the obesity problem is helped and the patient loses weight, the lifestyle that enabled the obesity is going to still be present. Using a natural remedy to reduce obesity enables you to keep slim and feeling good and balanced from the start.

Again, ScienceDaily.com summed it up well when they announced:

"For the first time, we have evidence that the amount of sleep makes a big difference on the results of dietary interventions. One should not ignore the way they sleep when going on a diet. Obtaining adequate sleep may enhance the beneficial effects of a diet. Not getting enough sleep could defeat the desired effects."

Two years later in 2012, ScienceDaily.com followed up with a related story entitled, *Lack of Sleep Makes Your Brain Hungry* in which they said this:

New research from Uppsala University shows that a specific brain region that contributes to a person's appetite sensation is more activated in response to food images after one night of sleep loss than after one night of normal sleep. Poor sleep habits can therefore affect people's risk of becoming overweight in the long run. [...]

In a new study, Christian Benedict, together with Samantha Brooks, Helgi Schiöth and Elna-Marie Larsson from Uppsala University and researchers from other European universities, have now systematically examined which regions in the brain, involved in appetite sensation, are influenced by acute sleep loss. By means of magnetic imaging (fMRI) the researchers studied the brains of 12 normal-weight males while they viewed images of foods. The researchers compared the results after a night with normal sleep with those obtained after one night without sleep. [...]

"After a night of total sleep loss, these males showed a high level of activation in an area of the brain that is involved in a desire to eat. Bearing in mind that insufficient sleep is a growing problem in modern society, our results may explain why poor sleep habits can affect people's risk to gain weight in the long run. It may therefore be important to sleep about eight hours every night to maintain a stable and healthy body weight."

The Rebuilding Hormone

DHEA[68] is an abbreviation for the hormone called *dehydroepiandrosterone*. Your adrenal gland produces DHEA. Like cortisol, DHEA is a stress hormone although DHEA and cortisol often find themselves working against each other as the way they handle stress differs.

DHEA could be considered a rebuilding hormone that begins to go to work when stress hits whereas cortisol does more damage when stress is present. This doesn't mean that cortisol is bad to have. The "damage" is a healthy damage that helps you eliminate some cell waste but too much cortisol certainly can be bad.

Combined with too little DHEA to help offset the damage; your body can get into trouble. As always you want all your hormones to work in harmony by being at their optimum balance levels.

Problems with DHEA Imbalance

Stress, anxiety, fear, and worry all contribute to DHEA (as well as cortisol and other hormone) imbalances. With normal levels of stress, offset by a good diet and moderate exercise, your DHEA levels to rise and then fall back when the stress dampens. Too much stress causes your body to increase production of cortisol at the expense of DHEA… producing too little of the rebuilding DHEA and too much of the tearing-down cortisol. The big problem is that your body might become incapable of reducing the cortisol levels or increasing your DHEA once the stress finally goes away.

Note: Another problem is that we tend to think of only one kind of stress. That is the stress that comes from life such as working too hard, worry, and so on. But physical accidents, surgery, and blood sugar changes cause your body to go through stress too. Your body responds the same way no matter what the stress source happens to be: DHEA and cortisol increases for a while to try to deal with the stress together but your DHEA gives up quickly and begins to drop to dangerously low levels while that cortisol just keeps on damaging.

You might have heard that prolonged stress makes you susceptible to disease and a DHEA imbalance is one of the key reasons why. Lowered DHEA (again, commonly accompanied with higher cortisol levels that don't drop properly) will put you at risk for all of the following problems:

- Immune system weakness

- Rising blood sugar levels

- Sodium and water retention

- High blood pressure

- Increased heart disease risk due to higher triglycerides

- Broken thyroid gland operation

- Increased belly fat

- Protein breakdown problems resulting in bone density problems

- There are more but need we go on? You want your DHEA in balance.

Too much DHEA over an extended period of time is rare except for people who over-supplement with DHEA. Acne is the primary side effect to watch for.

Putting Your DHEA in Balance

Guess what can cause a dangerous reduction in DHEA? Eating too many grains and having too much sugar. Guess what most people eat too much of?

If you've been a cereal and bread kind of person for as long as you can remember, and a salivary DHEA-cortisol test shows low levels of DHEA, before you worry about other corrective actions stop the grains *now*. Give yourself a month off grains and retest to see if there is any movement in your DHEA.

Allergies to various grains, such as wheat and rye, are far more prevalent than we used to think. Four decades of the government's FDA telling you to eat more grains than anything else will catch up to all of us eventually. It has caught up. The number of gluten and grain allergies is becoming an epidemic.

Oh, and long-term soy reduces the DHEA level in some people. Look in your kitchen cabinet at any package or can. Look at another. See how many list "soy" in some form or another. Then toss every one of those things in the garbage and go buy real food from a local farmer or farmer's market.

If your diet is good, then the chances are high that stress is the primary genesis of your low DHEA levels. Reducing your stress is the key. You do that through changing your lifestyle-related stress factors such as:

Getting more sleep, perhaps by supplementing with melatonin

Reducing your workload

Getting help dealing with family matters that may be causing strife

Sometimes stress factors that impact us are not in our control. So if you cannot reduce your lifestyle stress, and even if you can, you need to build up your body's resistance to stress. The way you do that is through exercise and diet. Adding fermented foods such as homemade kefir, yogurt, and cold-processed sauerkraut also help strengthen your family's resistance.

Good fats and proteins amplify your resistance to stress by enabling your body to respond strongly against stress. When flare-ups occur, a body that is more immune to that stress will deal with the stress, amplifying DHEA and cortisol together properly to help you reduce the stress's physical impact on you, and once reduced those levels will return to normal.

26
THE SEX-RELATED HORMONES

One of the most important aspects of hormonal balance comes to light in regards to sexual functioning.

Hormones are *everything* when it comes to sex drive with the rare exceptions of a physical (structural) problem or something internal such as endometriosis flaring up and making sex painful and unwanted. Of course emotional and relationship problems are often the cause of so many sexual problems, but surprisingly some of those can melt once one fixes internal hormonal problems such as estrogen or testosterone deficiencies or abundances.[69]

We'll focus primarily on these hormones next:

- Estrogen
- Progesterone
- Testosterone

Even if You Don't Miss the Sex

If you have no sex drive but you are happy with that and so is your spouse, or if you live alone and don't want a sex drive, you should understand that a healthy sex drive *is a sign of a healthy body* and the opposite is true also. No sex drive is often a major indicator of health problems. These problems often manifest themselves in sexual problems early before building to even more serious conditions later.

We're going to focus on a general state of healthiness and sexual function that typically accompany normal levels of the sexual hormones.

We're going to discuss what happens if you're too low or too high on those hormones and look for ways to balance them again. We're not going into all the ins and outs and possibilities simply because this is a vast region and for typical health and weight loss you just don't need the scientific depth that you can find elsewhere if you want that.

Sexual Supplements

Certainly supplements can play a major role in balancing the sex hormones. Unlike HGH and some others, sexual hormone supplements, through prescriptions, have been quite effective. (Some have been quite horrid too.) We won't ignore the supplementation issues, but given the focus of health and weight loss we will refer you to other sources for more in-depth and serious coverage of those issues.

So, now we'll focus on the balance of your sexual hormones and some of the more common and healthy ways to try to put them into balance through routine, healthy, natural methods.

The Sex Hormones for Women

In general, and this is only a rule of thumb, if you and your spouse love each other but have *any* problems sexually where disinterest of one party or the other is involved, then there is a brain nutrient or hormone problem. Yes, it can be emotional but hormones often trigger emotions that get blamed for such problems. Yes, it can be physical and it can be emotional and it's always wise to get everything checked. But assume that physical issues are not the primary blame until a professional determines otherwise.

For our purposes, a lack of desire and even physical pain of sex (such as endometriosis) can very well have origins in hormonal imbalances. Hormones determine your sex drive above all other factors.

Obviously estrogen is a primary female sex hormone that needs to be discussed, but healthy women also have low levels of testosterone (low relative to healthy men) and progesterone levels are also extremely critical. All three hormones need to be in balance for you, if female, to desire a healthy amount of sex. And a desire for sex is a primary sign of health so it's one that needs to be analyzed by a professional in almost every case. We'll work on fixing your hormones primarily by diet here, but you should also seek help from a nutritionally aware physician.

Menopause is Often a Problem Solved Badly

So many factors exist to consider that we have to narrow them down here to stay focused on your weight and general well-being. One of the most obvious evidences of a hormonal problem in women as they hit middle age is menopause. Menopausal women often find that their weight gain skyrockets and just gets out of control, perhaps for the first time in their lives.

If nothing has changed other than you've gotten older and your weight is up, you must remember that hormones affect your biochemistry directly. And the word *biochemistry* begins with *bio* and *bios* in Greek means *life*. The center of life's universe on earth is sex. That is where life begins and so that should be a primary focus of health. Don't shrug off menopausal weight gain or a growing lack of interest in sex as normal aging. Your very quality of *life* is on the line.

Many people, especially women, attack their aging weight problem with calorie-restrictive diets. As we've discussed before, restricting your calories does the following:

1. Makes you lose water weight quickly. (Almost *any* "diet" when followed will do this initially. That is why it's such as red herring making people believe they are following a good diet when it may be extremely dangerous as many calorie-restrictive diets are.)

2. Puts your body into long-term starvation mode, which puts your hormones in a tizzy like they've never seen before. This causes energy to be taken away from vital organs such as your liver in an attempt to keep you alive just a little longer after the lack of food for fuel.

3. Once you fall off the calorie-restriction diet, and you will, you gain the weight back and more due to your body's extreme craving at that moment for instant fuel that comes from horrible carbohydrates such as mashed potatoes, chips, bread, sweets, and other "comfort" foods that don't comfort your body but that do spike your body's blood sugar level.

Menopause itself comes about because of hormonal changes. You cannot stop it from happening of course, and you wouldn't want to if someone finds a way. Menopause is a normal function in a healthy life. But you can minimize the negatives and maximize your health in all other ways, including your weight, by understanding, which hormones are most susceptible and ways to work on normalizing them as much as possible.

Problems with Female Sex Hormone Imbalances

Aging affects the presence of a balance of female-related hormones such as estrogen and progesterone. If only aging was the only problem to deal with. Contraception can possibly disrupt your hormones, which is why you want to be checked carefully throughout your use of them. Caffeine affects your sex hormonal balance, as can alcohols and other sugars and starchy and sugary carbohydrates. Not surprisingly to these authors, fat-free dairy has been shown to be a major disruptor of female hormones.

So many things in the environment mimic hormones and estrogen mimicking is one of the worst culprits both for men and women.

Pesticides, soy, and preservatives in thousands of food products mimic the injection of our systems with substances that our bodies react to the same way they would react to excess estrogen production in our own glands.

Note: The World Health Organization, a governing body that seemingly wants more and more power if you look at its policies and recommendations, says that these parabens (estrogen look-a-likes) are low risk factors and can be ignored. The reason they state this is that parabens are up to 100,000 less potent than estrogen-related hormones so they pose little danger. That may very well be but what they fail to note is that these parabens appear in quantities up to *one million times the quantity of the estrogen-related hormones!*[70]) Therefore, by the WHO's own published standards, these estrogen-mimicking parabens are present at levels *ten times higher* than normal estrogen-like hormones factors. This poses a real danger to women. High estrogen levels are not always, and perhaps rarely, a result of the human body's own functioning. You need to be constantly aware of this as you buy your food. The next time you pass up organic produce, over conventional, consider the risks. These parabens also appear in heavy quantities in deodorants and guess what? Breast cancer often begins in the underarm areas! So you owe it to yourself to seek a natural deodorant for you and your family.

Increased estrogen exposure is most dangerous to children. Children as young as eight years old are experiencing puberty in record numbers over the past 2 decades. Why is that? Certainly it's not evolution. It has to be environmental.

By the way, *ginger* has properties shown to reduce this paraben toxicity according to a paper recently published by R.J. Verma from the University School of Sciences in Gujart University, India. As an added bonus, and a big bonus at that, ginger has incredible properties to maximize your brain's functioning.

For women, an imbalance of estrogen can portend serious issues such as:

- Weight gain (of course)
- Sexual dysfunction and desire issues
- Migraine headaches
- Tenderness in the breasts
- Infertility issues
- Uterine cancer
- Endometriosis
- Strokes
- Heart problems
- Decreased vaginal lubrication
- And this list is far from exhaustive.

The hormone progesterone is also a problem when it's out of balance even though it doesn't get the press that estrogen does. Progesterone helps regulate menstrual cycles, pregnancy, and embryo formation. In addition, progesterone works to help regulate estrogen. Again, here is an example of one hormone that needs to be in balance to help keep another hormone in balance. You cannot focus on single hormones in your body which is why we have tried to address the entire group through diet primarily first throughout this book.

- Progesterone imbalances can occur and when they do you may see signs of:
- Weight gain (of course); an over-abundance of estrogen can shift fat from your butt to your belly.
- Depression
- Period disruptions
- Menstrual problems such as excess bleeding
- Cysts in the breasts

Too large of a chest (that's possible even for women!) may be an indicator of progesterone problems.

A Doctor Weighs In

Recently, Dr. Joseph Mercola, MD, told his subscribers of the horrid impact of parabens and concluded with this, which we can find absolutely nothing to argue with:

Radically reduce your sugar/fructose intake. Normalizing your insulin levels by avoiding sugar and fructose is one of the most powerful physical actions you can take to lower your risk of cancer. Unfortunately, very few oncologists appreciate or apply this knowledge today. The Cancer Centers of America is one of the few exceptions, where strict dietary measures are included in their cancer treatment program. Fructose is especially dangerous, as research shows it actually speeds up cancer growth.

Optimize your vitamin D level. Ideally it should be over 50 ng/ml, but levels from 70-100 ng/ml will radically reduce your cancer risk. Safe sun exposure is the most effective way to increase your levels, followed by safe tanning beds and then oral vitamin D3 supplementation as a last resort if no other option is available.

Maintain a healthy body weight. This will come naturally when you begin eating right for your nutritional type and exercising using high-intensity burst-type activities[...]. It's important to lose excess weight because estrogen is produced in fat tissue.

Get plenty of high quality animal-based omega-3 fats, such as those from krill oil. Omega-3 deficiency is a common underlying factor for cancer.

Avoid drinking alcohol, or limit your drinks to one a day for women.

Breastfeed exclusively for up to six months. Research shows this will reduce your breast cancer risk.

Watch out for excessive iron levels. This is actually very common once women stop menstruating. The extra iron actually works as a powerful oxidant, increasing free radicals and raising your risk of cancer. So if you are a post-menopausal woman or have breast cancer you will certainly want to have your Ferritin level drawn. Ferritin is the iron transport protein and should not be above 80. If it is elevated you can simply donate your blood to reduce it.

By the way, high iron is also a problem for men and it often goes undetected due to men's common lack of requesting regular full-spectrum blood tests. Men never menstruate, and most don't get cuts and scrapes the way our forefathers who worked outdoors got. The best way for men to keep their iron levels at healthy levels also helps others: Men should give blood regularly. This is usually all that's needed to maintain a healthy level of iron.

Testosterone Isn't Just for Men

Women need testosterone to function normally just as men need some estrogen. The problem, as always, is balance.

If you have been showing signs of a low sex drive, obviously you need to begin the hormone-healthy diet lifestyle immediately, but you also need to get all your sexual hormone levels checked by a professional. Medical treatment of low levels of testosterone differs from that of, say, low levels of estrogen. (Fortunately, if diet alone will put your sexual functioning hormones back in balance, the same diet works well for all three: estrogen, progesterone, and testosterone. In addition, some other factors you'll learn about below will also help adjust them into better ranges.)

If your glands are producing too much testosterone, you could experience hair loss where you don't want it and hair growth where you don't want that! In addition your voice can deepen. Worse, you'll have a tendency to put on shoulder pads, try out for the team, and pat your teammates on the backside after each touchdown.

Note: We actually have no technical, scientific, or medical evidence that any of that last part will occur.

- Too little testosterone in women might at first seem to be a minor thing but the health problems related to low testosterone comprises a surprisingly complete list including:
- No sex drive and/or no orgasms
- Pain during sex
- Premature aging
- Depression and related disorders such as severe fear and depression
- Vaginal itching
- Muscle atrophy
- Low-fat diets can reduce your testosterone so stay away from those.

Putting Your Female Sex Hormones in Balance

First of all, a diet high in good fats goes a long way towards staving off these hormonal problems. Keep your protein up. A group of vegetables from the cruciferous family acts as both an estrogen-reducing agent and an antitoxin. These vegetables are all low in carbohydrates and include:

- Cabbage
- Broccoli
- Cauliflower
- Radish
- Kale
- Brussels sprouts

You must make a major inspection of your cosmetic sources as well as your food sources to help reduce the problems society finds itself having these days. Moving to a natural deodorant is a must and if you can find one without *any* aluminum (or alum) you will also keep more of that heavy metal from your system.

Green tea has some positive effects on female hormones.

Estrogen rarely is considered to be too low these days with all the hormone-mimicking estrogen, but it can occur. If you end up accepting a doctor's advice to get estrogen treatments, get a second opinion. If you then trust both opinions get bio-identical female hormone replacements. These *are* considered as safe as possible given the data we currently have. If it's not bio-identical, stay completely away as if it is pure poison.

Finally, a treatment that will make your husband jump for joy. More sex will increase your testosterone naturally. Obviously if you have pain then you might not be able to pursue this avenue until some of the other possible solutions kick in, but once you are able to you should begin trying sex once again… even if the desire isn't quite there yet. Go through the motions to help stimulate your testosterone levels and increase the speed at which your desire returns.

Note: Zinc is a good supplement for improving your sex hormone balances. Zinc plays a big role in fertility.

The Sex Hormones for Men

Men, certainly the hormone testosterone is a major hormone for you and the lifestyle you want to live. Testosterone literally defines you just as estrogen defines women. The thing you may not have known before is that your body, if healthy, also produces estrogen and progesterone. Your estrogen and progesterone levels, although far less than healthy levels for females are critical to keep in balance.

With aging brings a lowered sex drive naturally. That typically isn't a huge deal for men as long as the desire still remains and everything functions normally. If you begin to worry that things are no longer functioning normally, or if your desire seems to be far weaker than it has been in the distant past, then hormonal changes are almost certainly to be looked at.

Through a simple blood test doctors can check for your testosterone, estrogen, and progesterone levels. The results will let you know if one or more of those hormones are too weak or too strong.

It's true that the Erectile Dysfunction drugs have made a major impact on society today. It's also true that ED may very well be only a symptom and not a cause. Treating ED, when a symptom and not the cause, can rob you of a far more healthy *and active* life in all ways including sexually. The cause can often be, you guessed it, hormonal.

Problems with Male Sex Hormone Imbalances

Looking at testosterone first, abnormally low levels obviously can produce sexual dysfunction. Other than a gradual reduction due to aging, a more rapid decrease might signal a drop in testosterone production. You need to immediately fix your lifestyle to help the levels boost back up. (In severe drops, you may very well need hormone replacement therapy. Surprisingly, other than being somewhat costly without insurance, this treatment is fairly benign and has proved to work well in men.)

Not only will you have a lowered sex drive with lowered testosterone, you'll have the tendency to put on weight, especially around your middle stomach section. Middle age weight gain is not something you should focus on first as you now know well enough if you've read the book up to this point. You need to focus on your hormone levels first or you may never reduce that spare tire around your middle.

In addition to a low sex drive, erectile dysfunction, and weight gain, low testosterone levels can lead to:

- Looking far older than your actual age

- Indecisiveness

- Depression and related disorders such as anxiety and fear

- Decreased muscle mass which helps speed up your weight gain even further

- Wrinkles which aids in making you look even older than low testosterone already makes you look

Perhaps not surprisingly, the lack of confidence and indecisiveness may be why studies show women are more attracted to men with higher testosterone levels than low levels. If you get too much testosterone, you will experience these symptoms:

- Dramatically increased urination

- Enlarged prostate

- Baldness (baldness can occur naturally from regular healthy levels of testosterone due to genetics; bald uncles on your mother's side of the family are especially leading indicators that you have a natural tendency to lose hair more rapidly than you otherwise might)

Estrogen and Progesterone Aren't Just for Women Anymore

It's true that you men are not 100% raging testosterone machines. You are machines that, when healthy, also produce estrogen and progesterone and you need both of those, although in smaller quantities than testosterone.

When your estrogen levels are at high levels you can probably guess at the symptoms already. They are typically the opposite of a high testosterone situation and include:

- Abnormally large breasts (*manboobs*)
- Prostate trouble that leads to extreme urination frequencies
- Lowered sperm counts
- Higher voice
- Less facial and body hair
- Feminine characteristics in the way you project yourself

The problem with high estrogen levels is not usually that you produce too much. The problem is that it's the paraben-laced environment and your diet that can be, and often is, responsible for the feminization of men today from high estrogen levels. Through pesticides and an abundance of soy in almost every processed food that you eat, as well as an abundance of soy fed to cattle and chickens that were never designed to digest soy, you are getting tons of the stuff whether you want it or not.

Just as too little estrogen in men rarely occurs, fortunately too much progesterone occurs only in extremely rare cases. Most of the time an imbalance of progesterone in men occurs on the high side. This can affect your prostate negatively as well as give you symptoms of anxiety, excess fears, and nervousness.

Prostate Issues

It is said that:

Men either die of prostate problems or with prostate problems.

If you think about that for a bit, it seems as though prostate problems are inevitable and it's just a matter of when and how much. Although this may be true to some extent given the natural processes that occur in men as you age, it's almost always agreed that you don't have to die of prostate cancer in most cases. The easiest way is to avoid it altogether. The easiest way to do that is through diet. (You knew we would say that, right?)

Pumpkin seeds are good for keeping your prostate happy and eating them daily is never a bad thing. Buy organic.

Supplements can help ward off prostate problems too. It's widely known that saw palmetto (and nettle root which often comes with saw palmetto supplements) can help keep a prostate well but also omega-3 oils also work well towards keeping your prostate in good shape. In addition, the heart-healthy CoQ10 has been shown to have good effects on the prostate.

Putting Your Male Sex Hormones in Balance

It's easy to imagine Party Guy right? You know, he's the one who has a drink in one hand and a new girl in the other. The problem with that image, as college students sometimes find out in an embarrassing way, is that alcohol lowers your testosterone *and* raises your estrogen levels by causing a conversion of some testosterone to estrogen. Lower testosterone lowers your desirability in women as mentioned earlier. To compound this problem, alcohol also increases your stress hormone cortisol. And remember, higher cortisol levels and lower testosterone combine to cause women to be less attracted to men. So alcohol is a double-whammy for your sexual functioning.

> **Note:** You should emphasize eggs in your diet. Saturated fats and cholesterol-rich foods such as eggs play important roles in the production of sex hormones, especially for men. By the way, your body produces cholesterol. Your cholesterol doesn't increase with foods high in cholesterol no matter what the government's FDA has said for decades. 50% of heart attacks happen to people with "normal" cholesterol levels. Your brain *requires* cholesterol. While cholesterol can play a negative role when it's at extremely high levels, it isn't the bad guy it's made out to be. Many cultures have much higher levels of cholesterol than Americans, for example, yet have fewer heart attacks.

When Diet Isn't Enough

If diet alone doesn't seem to be enough, get a blood test to determine your testosterone, estrogen, and progesterone levels and see if more is needed. Supplements are available to help. B-complex vitamins are super and zinc specifically targets the sex hormones and seems to improve the levels.

With zinc, take about 100mg a day as a hormone-balancing supplement. Zinc inhibits the aromatase enzyme that converts testosterone to estrogen. You want that enzyme! At 100mg a day, zinc also helps block the conversion of your testosterone to DHT, which is a hormone that increases your chance to begin balding.

When it comes to testosterone replacement, it's actually fairly common and easy *and seems to be fairly safe* as long as your doctor monitors your levels. If you're middle age or older and you accept a natural testosterone replacement such as *Androgel,* there are some negative side effects, but they are rare and you want to be on the constant lookout that you don't start regaining too much testosterone. Too much can result in anger issues before you know it, at the regret of you and everybody around you later. Talk to your prescribing doctor about the problems that can occur and stay in contact every few months for a check to make sure that the levels you're prescribed are keeping you at the levels your physician approves of. Reducing or increasing the rate of application is supposed to be a minor adjustment so there's little reason not to maintain a proper level.

Note: One of the side effects most commonly written about, and that was actually made popular in an episode of the medical show *House*, is that anybody on hormone treatments such as testosterone replacement needs to make sure that he is the *only one getting the treatment!* In other words, you don't want to allow any part of your body where you apply the treatment to come in contact with other members of your family, wives *and children especially*, because testosterone can be transmitted from you to them. Generally, the patch or gel is applied to an area normally covered such as your shoulder area. Even a thin shirt is adequate. As long as you wash that area first, another family member such as your wife can put her head on your shoulder at night with no worry. But you need to know that this can be a major problem for your family if you don't monitor your place of contact.

Many of the modern testosterone replacement hormones are natural and not fully synthetic (these are not bio-identical though, like the good estrogen for women is). Still they appear to have excellent results with no statistical side effects. Monitor your blood levels closely the first few months and make sure you avoid direct skin contact with others in your family on the area where you apply the hormone.

27
THE ADRENALINE AND THE FIGHT OR FLIGHT HORMONES

Epinephrine, more commonly known as *adrenaline*,[71] is produced by your adrenal gland. Obviously epinephrine is a heart-related hormone because when you get excited or afraid, your heart rate rises and that's due to your body increasing your adrenaline to help prepare you for a fight-or-flight situation.

Epinephrine also helps to regulate other fight-or-flight factors such as breathing (by actually adjusting your air passage sizing) and your metabolism. When epinephrine (adrenaline) is pumping, your metabolism is in high gear too! Epinephrine also affects your liver, muscles, as well as your entire system.

Epinephrine is often used as a drug, especially under emergency conditions such as cardiac arrest. People who experience anaphylactic shock and high allergy risk patients are often given epinephrine to react to the attack and try to restore their bodies to a more normal state.

Note: Some people are severely allergic to fresh fish. They must carry an *EpiPen* (a ballpoint pen-like injection system that contains epinephrine) with them at all times in case they accidentally eat something that produces an allergic reaction. That reaction is often a severe restriction in her lungs and the "adrenaline-pumping" action of the epinephrine might very well be life-saving if this occurs.

Problems with an Epinephrine Imbalance

Obviously our focus isn't concerned with the trauma-related requirements of epinephrine.

Our focus here is getting and keeping our hormones in balance. Epinephrine has an effect on weight gain so it's worth knowing something about it and its cousin, norepinephrine.

Too much epinephrine causes you to gain weight. When your life is on the line, who cares about a massive injection of epinephrine? Otherwise you don't want to trigger an increase in epinephrine if you can help it.

Note: Anybody who has found themselves in the middle of a crime felt their adrenaline skyrocket. Afterwards they often find that they feel wobbly and weaker than they've ever felt. The dramatic epinephrine reduction after the event drains them to new low levels.

Putting Your Epinephrine in Balance

For one thing, stay away from typical diet pills to adjust your epinephrine!

Also, some people should watch their caffeine intake. Also, stay away from active crime scenes!

Seriously, the best way to avoid over-stimulating your own body with epinephrine is to keep your caffeine levels under control.

Note: Normally, pesticides are used at extreme levels when growing coffee beans. You are stacking up your hormonal disadvantages if you don't drink organic coffee.

Another Fight-or-Flight Hormone

Norepinephrine is a cousin to epinephrine.

Norepinephrine is also known as just *norepi*, *NE*, and *noradrenaline*. When your norepinephrine is elevated, your heart's contractions increase.

Norepinephrine usually appears in conjunction with epinephrine (adrenaline) in reaction to a fight-or-flight situation. The norepinephrine focuses on your heart the most, adjusting the heart's pumping action as needed. In addition to that, norepinephrine increases the blood to your muscles to prepare for whatever happens next as well as releases glucose from your cells for instant fuel.

All of this happens almost instantly in a healthy body when danger or extreme excitement arises (such as winning the lottery).

Problems with a Norepinephrine Imbalance

The problems of too much norepinephrine mirror those of too much epinephrine discussed in the previous chapter. Way too much caffeine is a common culprit. An upset in someone's production of norepinephrine in extreme cases can result in brain disorders including schizophrenia, depression, and severe ADD.

Putting Your Norepinephrine in Balance

Yep, everything on epinephrine holds true for norepinephrine. Reduce your caffeine if you're ingesting way too much (most people who drink a lot of coffee are fine).

There are ways to improve your norepinephrine balance. In general, you probably don't need to get tested for a norepinephrine imbalance barring some problem like a brain-related disease.

Instead, just do what you need to do daily to keep your norepinephrine and all your other hormones in good order. It shouldn't surprise you that the following foods are helpful for norepinephrine in particular:

- Eggs
- Meat
- Nuts

Yep, you heard all that before.

The very diet discussed in this section of the book, a good fat and good animal protein-based diet is good for norepinephrine just as it is the other hormones in your system.

Vitamin B6 can also help put norepinephrine and epinephrine back to good levels but you'll find B6 in beans, meat, chicken, and fish so there's little reason to supplement if you eat well.

The Additional Growth Hormone

The *insulin-like growth factor* hormone is often abbreviated *IGF-1*. It's also called *somatomedin C*. Your pituitary gland secrets IGF-1. From the name *insulin-like* growth hormone, you shouldn't be surprised to learn that IGF-1 is similar in structure to insulin.

IGF-1 called is secreted during our growing years so children can grow.

You want IGF-1 to be healthy if you're overweight because IGF-1 is a fat-burning hormone (along with HGH, glucagon, epinephrine, the thyroids T3 and T4, and testosterone).

Problems with an IGF-1 Imbalance

IGF-1 production naturally decreases as we age. We don't need the growth spurts we get in childhood and our activity levels naturally decrease as we age so our bodies don't produce as much IGF-1 because our bodies simply don't need the levels they once had. In spite of it being natural, the drawback of the slowing down of IGF-1 is that it ages us. Our cells break down and die, resulting in aging of our bodies.

If your pituitary gland begins to produce too little IGF-1, all of the following can begin to occur:

You gain weight

Your brain gets less blood impairing your critical thinking skills and causing you to react more slowly to stimuli; in addition to slowing your brain down your memory begins to fail and your IQ begins to suffer

Depression appears as well as related problems such as anxiety, fear, and severe mood swings with the low moods more common than the better moods

Your muscles begin to decrease

Your bone density decreases (Osteoporosis is helped along by a decrease in IGF-1 levels)

You are at a higher risk of heart disease, high blood pressure problems, and you can more easily take on a diabetic state

Your doctor can test you for growth hormone deficiencies including IGF-1 with a blood test. If your doctor doesn't see the need to do this but wants to treat your high blood pressure, diabetes symptoms, and depression with medicine before checking your HGH and IGF-1, get a second opinion from someone who understands the importance of balanced hormones.

Putting Your IGF-1 in Balance

A synthetic form of IGF-1 is available to help children who have FTT, *Failure to Thrive*... a growth condition where their bodies do not grow and mature normally.

For most of us, diet is the key. A high fat, high protein, smart carbs, no sugar lifestyle will go a long way towards restoring IGF-1 and related hormones.

Although you cannot stop the aging process, you certainly can speed it up through a bad diet. Focus on getting organic vegetables, grass-fed beef, cage-free poultry and eggs, and raw, whole milk to slow down the act of aging. Moderate exercise also seems to work to help stave off brain-related disorders and aspects of aging.

28
HORMONE SUMMARY

So there you have it. Fix your hormones if you want a healthy body and you want to be at your best weight. It works that way best. You'll rarely do your body much good if you work on your weight first. You will be working against yourself, going against the grain (did you catch that pun?). Your hormones simply won't let you lose weight and keep it off until you balance them.

Fix your hormone levels first and let them *help you* fix your body and weight.

So what are you waiting for? Ditch all your processed food, go *now* to get organic produce, grass fed beef, cage-free chicken and eggs, raw, whole milk, and lots of good oils and nuts and seeds.

The core thing to remember is that if you are having problems losing weight and feeling energetic even though you "eat well" and exercise a lot, then maybe diet and exercise aren't the most important problems holding you back from losing weight and feeling great. If you feel bad or are overweight... the problem is most likely a hormonal imbalance.

29
1-DAY DIET CONCLUSION

The 1-Day Diet book is in essence three books in one. The first section describes the lead diet... *The 1-Day Diet*. If you want to lose weight as fast as possible while saving money in the process, you're all set. As long as you follow the outline, it's totally safe and extremely healthy for you to do. The great thing is, you can go on and off the *1-Day Diet* for the rest of your life at your convenience.

The 1-Day Diet works well by itself and together with the *5:2 Diet* (the second section of this book) and another of our diets, *The 10-Hour Coffee Diet*. http://www.amazon.com/10-Hour-Coffee-Diet-Transform-Health-ebook/dp/B00HB77U44/

In the third section of this book we talk about hormones and the major role they play in health and weight loss. Even though hormones and your diet work together, it's important for people to sometimes take a step back from looking at fixing their weight through diet-eyes. I hope we were able to get you to see things through "hormone-eyes" because fixing your health, and hormones, first will then lead to weight loss and a better body.

Good luck and we hope to hear about your weight loss and health transformation. We'd be grateful if you could share your results and thoughts (both good and bad) of the 1-Day Diet book by writing a review on Amazon.

Here are the links to the book page on Amazon USA and Amazon UK:

http://www.amazon.com/1-Day-Diet-Fastest-World-ebook/dp/B005DR6LJE

and

http://www.amazon.co.uk/1-Day-Diet-Fastest-World-ebook/dp/B005DR6LJE

Sincerely,

Jennifer Jolan and Rich Bryda

P.S. If you're on Facebook you can find us here:

https://www.facebook.com/ 10HourCoffeeDiet

BONUS GIFTS!

As a special thank you for buying this book, you can get the following 10 reports *free* at our website: http://WeightLossEbookStore.com/

1. *How to Lose Weight Spinning in a Circle like Kids*
2. *The 20-Second Bathroom Trick for a Super-Charged Metabolism and a Flood of Energy*
3. *One Tablespoon of this $6 Supplement Detoxes 900 Yards of Toxins from Your Body*
4. *Do-It-Yourself Face-Lift: How to Look 5 Years Younger in 2 Weeks – Got 5 Minutes a Day?*
5. *The 50-Cent Miracle Weight Loss Food You're Not Eating*
6. *#1 Cheap Supplement that Reverses Gray Hair & Infuses Health into Your Body*
7. *How to Get Rid of Allergies in 90 Seconds with Water*
8. *The Ultimate 3-Second Fountain of Youth "Neural" Fat Loss Exercise*
9. *The 15-Second "T-Tap" for Overcoming Hypothyroidism & Sluggish Energy*
10. *How to Make Healthy Ice Cream in 2 Minutes and Other Sweet Surprises!*

REFERENCES

[1] *"Could you be losing muscle instead of fat? (Here's how not to do that!),"* https://www.pacifichealthlabs.com/blog/could-you-be-losing-muscle-instead-of-fat-heres-how-not-to-do-that/

[2] *"Basic Metabolic Rate – BMI / BMR Calculator,"* http://www.bmi-calculator.net/bmr-calculator/

[3] *"Needing advice about fasting options, please,"* http://www.myfitnesspal.com/topics/show/878853-needing-advice-about-fasting-options-please

[4] *"Intermittent Fasting Finally Becoming Mainstream Health Recommendation,"* http://fitness.mercola.com/sites/fitness/archive/2013/01/18/intermittent-fasting-approach.aspx

[5] *"Insulin and leptin as adiposity signals,"* http://www.ncbi.nlm.nih.gov/pubmed/14749506

[6] *"Hormone Ghrelin Raises Desire for High-Calorie Foods,"* http://www.webmd.com/diet/news/20100622/hormone-ghrelin-ups-desire-for-high-calorie-foods

[7] *"Human Growth Hormone (HGH),"* http://www.webmd.com/fitness-exercise/human-growth-hormone-hgh

[8] *"Triglycerides: Why do they matter?,"* http://www.mayoclinic.org/diseases-conditions/high-blood-cholesterol/in-depth/triglycerides/ART-20048186

[9] *"Free-radical theory of aging,"* http://en.wikipedia.org/wiki/Free-radical_theory_of_aging

[10] *"What Is Inflammation? What Causes Inflammation?,"* http://www.medicalnewstoday.com/articles/248423.php

[11] *"Insulin Sensitivity,"* http://www.diabetes.co.uk/insulin/insulin-sensitivity.html

[12] *"Type 2,"* http://www.diabetes.org/diabetes-basics/type-2/

[13] *"The 10-Hour Coffee Diet,"* http://www.amazon.com/10-Hour-Coffee-Diet-Transform-Health-ebook/dp/B00HB77U44/

[14] *"Tyrosine Overview Information,"* http://www.webmd.com/vitamins-supplements/ingredientmono-1037-TYROSINE.aspx?activeIngredientId=1037&activeIngredientName=TYROSINE

[15] *"Green Tea Extract, Thermogenis-Induced Weight Loss,"* http://www.ncbi.nlm.nih.gov/pubmed/17201629

[16] *"What Are Xenoestrogens and How Do They Make You Fat?,"* http://www.healthline.com/health-blogs/hold-that-pause/what-are-xenoestrogens-fat"

[17] *"Beyond BPA: Why to Avoid Plastic Food Containers,"* http://www.thekitchn.com/beyond-bpa-why-to-avoid-plasti-140736

[18] *"Warm Lemon Water: A Natural Diuretic and Toxin Remover,"* http://consciouslifenews.com/warm-lemon-water-natural-diuretic-toxin-remover/

[19] *"Cinnamon Can Help Lower Blood Sugar, But One Variety May Be Best,"* http://www.npr.org/blogs/thesalt/2013/12/30/255778250/cinnamon-can-help-lower-blood-sugar-but-one-variety-may-be-best

[20] *"Use Cinnamon to Improve Insulin Sensitivity,"* http://www.muscleforlife.com/use-cinnamon-to-improve-insulin-sensitivity/

[21] *"Cinnamon boosts brain activity,"* http://www.nutraingredients.com/Research/Cinnamon-boosts-brain-activity

[22] *"Why Soy is Bad for You,"* http://www.optimumchoices.com/Soy.htm

[23] *"Soy Bad, Soy Good: The Pluses of Fermented Soy,"* http://articles.mercola.com/sites/articles/archive/2004/08/04/fermented-soy.aspx

[24] *"Running Sucks!,"* http://www.amazon.com/Running-SUCKS-Fast-Weight-Loss-ebook/dp/B005CWJJ6C

[25] http://www.oism.org

[26] *"Stevia: The 'Holy Grail' of Sweeteners?,"* http://articles.mercola.com/sites/articles/archive/2008/12/16/stevia-the-holy-grail-of-sweeteners.aspx

[27] http://www.choosemyplate.gov/

[28] *"Don't Drink Your Fruit,"* http://www.independentlivingnews.com/2013/10/09/shocking-report-fruit-juice-fat/

[29] *"Sodium benzoate is a preservative that promotes cancer and kills healthy cells,"* http://www.naturalnews.com/033726_sodium_benzoate_cancer.html

[30] *Journal of Applied Toxicology* , March, 2012, pgs. 219-232.

[31] http://nusi.org/about-us/a-letter-from-the-founders/gary-taubes/

[32] *"Food 101: Why Wild Alaskan Salmon Is Much Safer Than Farmed Salmon,"* http://blog.diginn.com/2012/06/26/food-101-why-wild-alaskan-salmon-is-much-better-for-you-than-farmed-salmon/

[33] *"Trans fat,"* http://en.wikipedia.org/wiki/Trans_fat

[34] *"Increasing Health and Immunity with Tropical Oils,"* http://www.jennette-turner.com/publications.cfm?id=7

[35] http://www.westonaprice.org/

[36] *"Why Counting Calories Doesn't Work,"* http://www.cbn.com/health/nutrition/drlen_countcalories.aspx

[37] *Facts about Diabetes and Insulin,* http://www.nobelprize.org/educational/medicine/insulin/diabetes-insulin.html

[38] *"The process of oxidation in the human body,"* http://www3.amherst.edu/~dmirwin/Reports/BetterHealth.htm

[39] *"Immune System, NIAID, NIH - National Institutes of Health,"* http://www.niaid.nih.gov/topics/immunesystem/Pages/default.aspx

[40] http://io9.com/5979523/why-you-should-starve-yourself-a-little-bit-each-day

[41] http://fitness.mercola.com/sites/fitness/archive/2013/03/01/daily-intermittent-fasting.aspx

[42] *"Fatty Liver Disease,"* http://www.webmd.com/hepatitis/fatty-liver-disease

[43] *"Metabolic Disorders: MedlinePlus,"* http://www.nlm.nih.gov/medlineplus/metabolicdisorders.html

[44] *"Fasting - Royal Road To Health And Long Life,"* http://www.webnat.com/articles/Fasting.asp

[45] *"Paul Dudley White,"* http://en.wikipedia.org/wiki/Paul_Dudley_White

[46] *Weston A. Price Foundation,* http://www.westonaprice.org/

[47] http://www.theiflife.com/

[48] http://articles.mercola.com/sites/articles/archive/2013/04/24/tea-bags.aspx

[49] *"Think Spice: 8 Spices with Health Benefits,"* http://www.fitnessmagazine.com/recipes/healthy-eating/superfoods/healthy-spices/

[50] *"Thermic effect of food,"* http://en.wikipedia.org/wiki/Thermic_effect_of_food

[51] *"TERRY WAHLS, M.D. The Wahls Protocol™: How I Beat Progressive MS,"* http://www.terrywahls.com/

[52] "Endocrine System," http://www.innerbody.com/image/endoov.html

[53] *Vegetables without Vitamins," Life Extension Magazine,* March 2001.

[54] *"GMO Facts,"* http://www.nongmoproject.org/learn-more/

[55] *"Incredible Egg!,"* http://www.incredibleegg.org/egg-facts/eggcyclopedia/h/hormones

[56] "Why lard's healthier than you think," http://www.thestar.com/life/health_wellness/nutrition/2013/05/14/why_lards_healthier_than_you_think.html

[57] "Why do potatoes raise blood glucose more than sugar?," http://lowcarbdiets.about.com/od/questionsandanswers/a/potatoglycemic.htm

[58] Walton Feed website, http://waltonfeed.com/

[59] "Thyroid Hormone," http://en.wikipedia.org/wiki/Thyroid_hormone

[60] "Hypothyroidism (underactive thyroid)," http://www.mayoclinic.org/diseases-conditions/hypothyroidism/basics/definition/CON-20021179

[61] "Digestive Disorders Health Center," http://www.webmd.com/digestive-disorders/picture-of-the-pancreas

[62] Dr. Berg Blog, http://www.drberg.com/blog/weight-loss/exercise-to-trigger-fat-burning-hormones

[63] "The role of glucagon in the body," http://www.diabetes.co.uk/body/glucagon.html

[64] Long Term Weight Loss for Thyroid Patients: Hormonal Factors That Affect Diets, http://thyroid.about.com/od/loseweightsuccessfully/a/weight-loss-diet.htm

[65] "Melatonin – Overview," http://www.webmd.com/sleep-disorders/tc/melatonin-overview

[66] "Cortisol Imbalance Symptoms," http://www.livestrong.com/article/94310-cortisol-imbalance-symptoms/

[67] "What is serotonin? What does serotonin do?," http://www.medicalnewstoday.com/articles/232248.php

[68] "DHEA," http://www.mayoclinic.org/drugs-supplements/dhea/background/HRB-20059173

[69] "Sexual desire and your hormones," http://www.netdoctor.co.uk/womenshealth/features/sexualdesire.htm

[70] The Journal of Applied Toxicology, March, 2012

[71] "What is Epinephrine?," http://www.news-medical.net/health/What-is-Epinephrine-(Adrenaline).aspx

53593745R00099

Made in the USA
Middletown, DE
28 November 2017